Color Atlas of

PEDIATRIC ENDOCRINOLOGY AND GROWTH

Color Atlas of

PEDIATRIC ENDOCRINOLOGY AND GROWTH

Jeremy K. H. Wales
Senior Lecturer in Pediatric Endocrinology
The University Department of Pediatrics
Sheffield Children's Hospital
Sheffield, UK

Alan D. Rogol
Professor of Pediatrics and Pharmacology
Chief, Division of Endocrinology and Metabolism
Children's Medical Center
Charlottesville
Virginia, USA

Jan Maarten Wit
Professor of Pediatrics
University Hospital
Leiden, The Netherlands

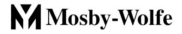

London Baltimore Barcelona Bogotá Boston Buenos Aires Caracas Carlsbad, CA Chicago Madrid Mexico City Milan Naples, FL New York
Philadelphia St. Louis Seoul Singapore Sydney Taipei Tokyo Toronto Wiesbaden

Copyright © 1996 Times Mirror International Publishers Limited

Published in 1996 by Mosby-Wolfe, an imprint of Times Mirror International Publishers Limited

Printed by Grafos S.A. Arte sobre papel, Barcelona, Spain.

ISBN 0 7234 2137 4

For full details of all Times Mirror International Publishers Limited titles, please write to Times Mirror International Publishers Limited, Lynton House, 7–12 Tavistock Square, London WC1H 9LB, England.

A CIP catalogue record for this book is available from the British Library.

Library of Congress Cataloging-in-Publication Data applied for.

Project Manager:	Jeremy Theobald
Developmental Editor:	Jennifer Prast
Cover Design:	Lara Last
Illustration:	Paul Bernson
Production:	Jane Tozer
Index:	Nina Boyd
Publisher:	Richard Furn

Contents

Acknowledgements   vii

Preface   ix

Key to Growth Charts and Interpretation of Clues   xi

Chapter 1
History, Auxology and Examination   1

Chapter 2
The Short Child   33

Chapter 3
The Large Child   67

Chapter 4
Early Sexual Development   81

Chapter 5
Late Sexual Development   93

Chapter 6
Abnormal Genitalia   99

Chapter 7
Goiter   117

Chapter 8
Abnormal Laboratory Values   125

Suggested Reference List   143

Appendix A
Tests of Endocrine Function   147

Appendix B
Normal Values   155

Index   159

Acknowledgements

Mr MJ Bell
Prof RM Blizzard
Dr CR Buchanan
Dr JM Buckler
Dr PE Clayton
Dr M Cork
Dr H Davies
Mr RB Fraser
Dr AT Gibson
Dr M Jansen
Dr MS Kibirige
Mr AE Mackinnon

Prof RDG Milner
Dr D O'Neill
Dr W Oostdijk
Dr RG Pearse
Mrs M Pickering
Dr B Rikken
Prof M Saleh
Dr A Sprigg
Dr RG Stanhope
Prof JL Van den Brande
Dr WG Wilson

Mr J Burke, Mr IM Strachan and the Orthoptic Department, Sheffield Children's Hospital
The Medical Illustration Departments at Sheffield, Leiden, Utrecht, Charlottesville and the Great Ormond Street Hospital for Sick Children NHS Trust.

Preface

Pediatric endocrine and growth disorders lend themselves to a problem-oriented approach to diagnosis. They are also often associated with clinical signs that may be demonstrated photo- and radiographically. Children are growing beings and their growth charts also provide a wealth of information. We have collected together prime illustrations of examples of these disorders from two continents in a book that is designed as a manual for the primary care physician and the non-specialist. The text aims to give guidance for the diagnosis of endocrine and growth disorders and to allow referral to the appropriate local specialist for further diagnostic evaluation and management. We hope that specialist pediatric and adult endocrinologists and physicians in training will be able to use the book as a teaching resource.

Each chapter has a common lay-out, setting out brief details of physiology, a diagnostic classification, a work-up (including history, examination and investigations) together with a brief plan of management. Space does not allow for a detailed description of endocrine anatomy or biochemistry and the interested reader is referred to one of the excellent comprehensive texts on the subject (p 143).

Much endocrine therapy is highly specialized and the focus of active research and debate. We have restricted our descriptions to well-established treatments, but also indicated areas of controversy. There is a large overlap of pediatric endocrinology with clinical genetics. As it would be impossible to illustrate even a minority of clinical syndromes, particularly those associated with short stature, we have tried to outline a broad diagnostic approach rather than give specific details, except in the most common and most important examples.

We believe that the atlas is comprehensive and that it approaches some of the goals we set out to achieve. We are grateful to colleagues in the United Kingdom, the Netherlands and the United States of America, some of whom are detailed on the previous page, for their assistance and support and, of course, to the patients whose photographs and data form the bulk of the work.

KEY TO GROWTH CHARTS

All the growth charts shown in this book utilize the same symbols, as follows:

•——	= Height
○- - -	= Bone age TW2-RUS
☐- - -	= Bone age G & P
X	= Final height prediction

TH = Target height, calculated in centimeters as follows:

$$Ht(boy) = \frac{[Ht(father) + Ht(mother) + 12]}{2} \qquad Ht(girl) = \frac{[Ht(mother) + Ht(father) - 12]}{2}$$

In imperial units, measure height in inches and apply a correction of ±4.75 inches.

A correction of +3 cm (+1½ inches) has been added to the target height to allow for secular trends.

The bottom panel shows the change in height standard deviation score (see text) with age.

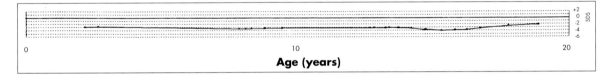

Age (years)

KEY TO INTERPRETATION OF CLUES

Throughout the book various combinations of signs, symptoms and investigations may indicate the strong likelihood of a particular diagnosis. This has been indicated by an = sign. Please bear in mind that there is always room for uncertainty in any diagnosis and it is rare for the *most likely* diagnosis to represent the *only possible* diagnosis.

1.
History, Auxology and Examination

HISTORY

All diagnosis begins with a comprehensive history and examination. This chapter will cover general points in the assessment of a child who may have an endocrine disorder. More specific points will be included in subsequent sections.

First, explore in detail the presenting complaint as perceived by the parents. If the patient is old enough ask if *he or she* has any concerns, or establish if this is a problem only to other family members or medical personnel.

Take details of the pregnancy (including ill-health or drug administration), the gestational age, mode of delivery and any requirement for neonatal special care. Usually, every mother can recall the birth weight of her offspring. It may be possible to obtain birth length and head-circumference from parental or hospital records. It is important to obtain information regarding rates of growth in height and weight as recorded in past medical records or perceived by the parents and child. Has there been recent gain or loss of weight? Is the child growing out of his or her clothes and shoes before they wear out?

Establish a family tree that records details of the heights (preferably measured directly), build and age of sexual maturation of both parents, siblings and any

more distant relations of aberrant stature. Inquire if there is parental consanguinity that may lead to an increased risk of autosomal recessive disorders. Ask if there are any family members with ill health, especially autoimmune (rheumatoid, pernicious anemia, alopecia, vitiligo) or 'gland' problems and then specifically inquire about thyroid disorders and insulin-dependent diabetes mellitus. The pedigree can be used to record social details that may be vitally important when considering both etiology and subsequent treatment and prognosis (**1.1**).

Is the patient on any regular medication (including topical and inhaled preparations)? Ask about past medical events including even what might be perceived as minor surgical procedures such as hernia repair or orchidopexy. Inquire about the current and early diet, and any specific exclusions.

Depending on the age of the child, establish the developmental or educational level and ask about the ability to participate actively in sport. Is there any bullying from peers? In the adolescent ask about career plans. Finally, run through the other systems of the body not involved in the presenting complaint to exclude other pathology.

The main points that must be established from the history of a child presenting with an endocrine disorder are given in **1.2**.

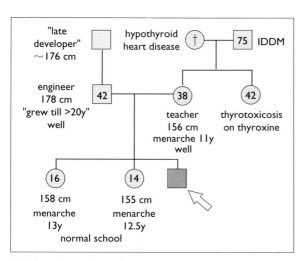

1.1 Family growth pedigree.

Essential points in the history

Details of presenting problem and level of concern
Details of mother's pregnancy and of delivery
Birth weight/other neonatal measurements if available
Family sizes, age at sexual maturity
Family history of endocrine or autoimmune disease
Social details
Medication, by any route
Past illnesses or operations
Diet in infancy and current intake
Current growth out of clothes/shoes – any past formal
    records of growth
Developmental or educational level
Bullying/peer pressure
Any specific symptoms in chest/CVS/GI/CNS/skin?

1.2 Essential points in the history.

AUXOLOGY

Detailed measurements can give an immense amount of information when properly performed and charted. Ideally, both parents should have measurements of at least height and weight recorded directly, since reported size can vary greatly from reality.

WEIGHT

This is a deceptively simple measurement that is often performed very badly. An infant should be weighed naked (**1.3**) and a child in the minimal clothing compatible with modesty (**1.4**). A modern disposable diaper can weigh as much as 0.45 kg (1 lb) when wet and the indoor clothing of a child wearing sports shoes and jeans weighs around 1.5 kg (3 lb 5 oz). These weights compare with a mean bodyweight gain in mid-childhood of 2–3 kg ($4\frac{1}{2}$–$6\frac{1}{2}$ lb per year). All scales should be regularly calibrated and serviced. The approximate weight of a struggling child can be deduced by weighing in the mother's arms followed by subtraction of the maternal weight.

LENGTH OR HEIGHT

Under the age of two, and in children with motor disability, it is usual to record supine length (**1.5**). This requires two people, often the mother plus auxologist. The head is held against the headboard with the face in a horizontal plane. The hips and knees are gently extended whilst keeping the pelvis horizontal and the movable foot board brought up to touch the soles of the feet held at 90°.

Standing height (**1.6**) should be measured using a stadiometer or other rule, in bare feet with the heels in the same vertical plane as the measuring instrument. The arms should be held relaxed at the sides, and the face should be in the 'Frankfurt plane' with the outer canthus of the eye and the external auditory meatus horizontal. The subject should be asked to take a deep breath in, then out whilst the auxologist exerts gentle upward traction on the mastoid processes. Height is read to the nearest completed millimeter at the end of the breath. If repeated measurements of height are taken to establish a growth velocity then, ideally, they should be performed at the same time of day to avoid errors due to spinal compression. (On average the height measured in the morning is 8 mm [$\frac{1}{3}$ inch] more than the afternoon value.) The standard error of measurement of height on a single occasion in the hands of a trained auxologist is in the order of 0.25 cm.

CROWN–RUMP LENGTH OR SITTING HEIGHT

The estimation of the length of the back and head can be of great benefit in establishing the relative proportions of the body. In an infant the legs are drawn up to 90° and the foot board brought into contact with the buttocks (**1.7**). In an older child, using a specially designed instrument (**1.8**) with the feet resting on a bar, the arms folded loosely in the lap and a

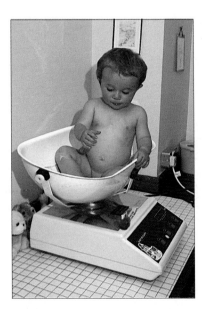

1.3 Measurement of infant weight. The nappy is removed and the calibration checked frequently.

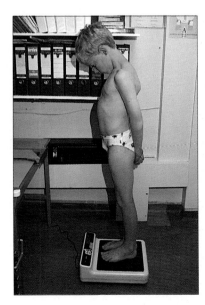

1.4 Measurement of weight. Minimal clothing on calibrated electronic scales.

similar stretch technique to the one described above, it is possible to obtain precise estimates of sitting height. A simpler method uses a hard seat of known height and horizontal top placed under the height stadiometer. Crown–rump length or sitting height may then be subtracted from standing height to derive sub-ischial leg length.

HEAD CIRCUMFERENCE

A non-stretchable paper or metal tape measure should be used and three measurements made of the maximum occipitofrontal circumference (OFC) (**1.9**). In children with abnormal head shape it may not be possible to obtain accurate readings.

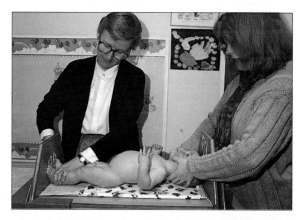

1.5 Measurement of infant length. Mother used to position head horizontally, auxologist gently to extend legs.

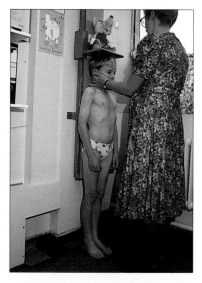

1.6 Measurement of height using stretch technique. Child in bare feet, using wall mounted stadiometer.

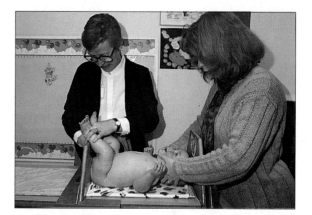

1.7 Measurement of infant crown–rump length.

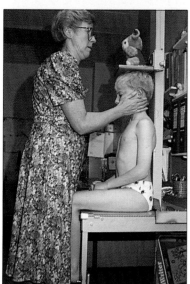

1.8 Measurement of sitting height. Stretch technique, using purpose built sitting height table.

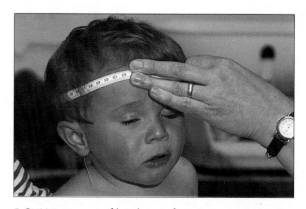

1.9 Measurement of head circumference using non-stretchable tape measure.

SKINFOLD THICKNESSES

A skinfold calliper is required that has a known strength of pinch and a known area of tip. Four sites are often chosen, of which the first two are in most common use. The triceps skinfold (**1.10**) is determined with the left arm loose at the side and a fold raised between the measurer's thumb and forefinger at the mid-point of the dorsum of the upper arm. The callipers are applied and after the reading has stabilized (4 or 5 seconds), the reading is made. The sub-scapular skinfold (**1.11**) is raised at the tip of the shoulder blade, on the left, with the arms again relaxed at the sides. The biceps skinfold (**1.12**) is determined as for the triceps skinfold but on the ventral aspect of the upper arm. The supra-iliac fold (**1.13**) is found at the maximum height of the iliac crest. Skinfold thicknesses give an estimation of the amount of subcutaneous fat and its distribution, and may be used in various equations to estimate total body adiposity. Centile charts can be used to demonstrate changes in fat thickness with therapy.

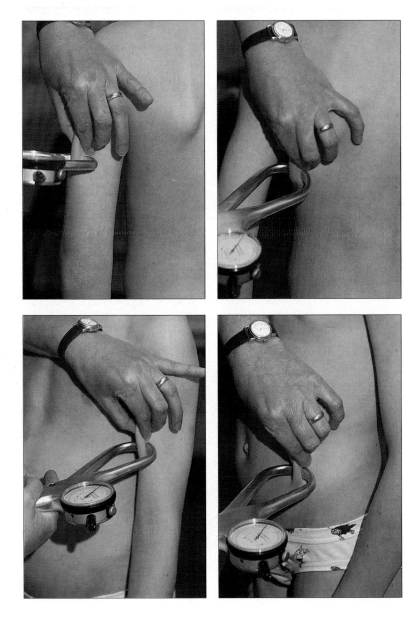

1.10–1.13 Measurement of triceps (left), biceps (lower left), subscapular (right) and supra-iliac (lower right) skinfold thickness.

BODY MASS INDEX

Another commonly used estimate of relative obesity is the body mass index (or Quetelet index), which can be estimated from the formula:

$$\frac{weight\,(kg\,)}{height\,(m\,)^2}$$

OTHER MEASUREMENTS

It is sometimes helpful to assess other body measurements and their relationships directly. Standard centile charts exist for almost every imaginable parameter. A measurement of span is the most likely to be of use in the endocrine clinic and may be estimated by measuring the fingertip to fingertip distance with the arms held horizontally (**1.14**). The normal relationship of span to height is:

span = height ± 3.5 cm (1½ in).

In short limbed conditions and if hemihypertrophy is suspected (see below), then direct measurement of limb segments using a specially designed anthropometer (**1.15**) or a builder's metal tape-measure may be of help.

GROWTH CHARTS

Up to date standards for height, weight and head circumference are available for many populations. Standards should be up-dated regularly to take secular changes in growth into account, and ideally ethnic sub-groups should be compared to appropriate charts, though this is not always possible.

Standards for sitting height, leg length, skinfold thickness, body mass index, span etc are less universally available, but published.

Most commonly used charts are sex-specific and show the measured parameter on the vertical axis and age on the horizontal. Almost all scales are linear except for skinfold thickness, where a vertical logarithmic axis is used, and in some charts extending into premature infancy, where a non-linear age axis allows expansion of data in the early months.

Charts of height and weight in many, named syndromic conditions have been published and should be used where necessary. There are also charts of limb length, height and OFC for many of the skeletal dysplasias.

The measured value should be plotted as a simple dot and other values, such as bone age (see below), plotted in a different color or as a square symbol or open circle (i.e. as per the key on page ix).

Whenever a standard centile chart is used, of whatever construction, it is possible to estimate rapidly the expected genetic potential of the subject by plotting the centile value of each parent on the right-hand *y* axis. The mid-parental centile can then be drawn. Alternatively, for height only, the following simple calculations of target height may be performed (where Ht = height in cm):

$$Ht\,(boy\,) = \frac{[\,Ht\,(father\,) + Ht\,(mother\,) + 12\,]}{2}$$

$$Ht\,(girl\,) = \frac{[\,Ht\,(mother\,) + Ht\,(father\,) - 12\,]}{2}$$

(or, in imperial units, height in inches plus a correction of 4 inches).

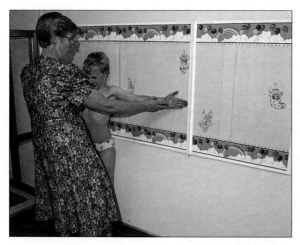

1.14 Measurement of span. The arms are horizontal, with the right finger tips held against a fixed vertical bar and the left against a movable vertical guide on calibrated graph paper.

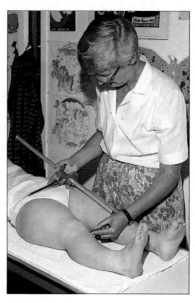

1.15 Measurement of individual body segments in a child with short limbs, using an anthropometer.

If a secular trend is expected, for example if the economic situation of the child is much better than that of the parents in their youth, one can add 3 cm (approximately 1 inch) to the target height. In 95% of the cases the final height of the child is expected to be within the target height ± 9 cm (3½ inches), the so-called 'target range'. The centile position of the target height can than be compared to the centile position of the present height of the child. This is the method used in illustrations throughout this book.

As growth is a longitudinal process, change of height with time is even more important than absolute height at a point. The final evaluation of growth in any parameter is made by connecting consecutive measurements on the growth chart and visually assessing any deviation upwards or downwards through the centile lines.

Growth rate can also be evaluated by calculating a velocity that can be compared with published height (and weight) velocity curves. Velocity is calculated by the formula:

$$\frac{Ht\,2 - Ht\,1}{Interval\;(years)}$$

Because measurement error is magnified when two separately obtained values are used to calculate a velocity (95% confidence interval (CI) for velocity estimated from two measurements one year apart = ± [2 SD of measurement (around 0.25 cm)] x √2; for a three month interval the CI is 4 times this value), the use of this calculation is dependent on accurate measurements and improved by long intervals between estimates. The design of the reference charts means that optimal information will come from yearly estimations of height velocity (and in clinical practice minimum periods of six months).

To allow more precise quantification of any normally distributed parameter for which standards exist it is common to use the Standard Deviation Score (SDS or Z-score), especially for values that lie outside the normal centile range. This technique allows comparison of the parameters for children of different age and sex.

$$SDS = \frac{x - \bar{x}}{SD}$$

(Where x is the measured value, x̄ is the mean and SD the standard deviation for a given population of that age and sex.)

In a normally distributed population, the SDS will have a mean of 0 and a SD of 1. A SDS of -1 to +1 includes 68.26% and one of -2 to +2 includes 95.44% of the population, respectively. Only 0.13% of a population will have a SDS of more or less than 3. The 0.4th centile may also sometimes be used to indicate extremes of 'normality'.

EXAMINATION

The examination of the child can begin during the history-taking by observing activity, demeanor and interaction with the parents or carers. It is then usual to begin with the hands, work up the arms to the head and neck, examine the chest and back, then the cardiovascular system followed by the abdomen and external inspection of the genitalia with an assessment of maturity. Finish with the central nervous system examination and inspection of the body and skin. These points are now described in more detail.

THE HANDS

The hands (and, sometimes, the feet) hold the clue to many endocrine disorders and syndromic malformations associated with abnormal stature. **1.16** through to **1.45** show a number of abnormalities and their interpretations.

Abnormal dermatoglyphics (**1.16**) such as a single palmar crease are non-specific signs of possible syndromic malformations. The fingers and wrist may be conveniently used to demonstrate increased mobility (**1.17**, **1.18**), as may be seen in the Marfan syndrome and some of the collagen disorders, or stiffness in long-standing diabetes mellitus (**1.19**) and some of the storage disorders (**1.20**, **1.21**). The skin may be thickened and stiff, producing joint immobility, in several syndromes associated with short stature (**1.22**). Fixed joint contractures (arthrogryposis) (**1.23**) may be restricted to one group of joints, or may be generalized. It is a non-specific sign of congenital neuromuscular disease and various syndromes. Long, thin fingers (arachnodactyly) are seen in the Marfan syndrome (**1.24**, **1.25**) and generally

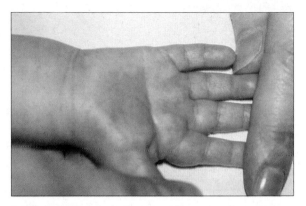

1.16 Single palmar crease – may be a normal variant but can be a non-specific clue to look for other dysmorphic features.

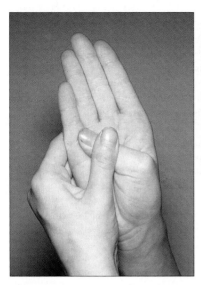

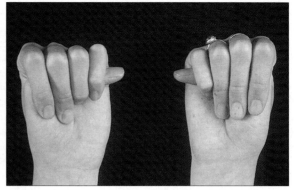

1.17, 1.18 Increased joint mobility in Marfan syndrome shown by touching palm with length of thumb (left) and ability to enclose thumb, which protrudes from the other side, with the clenched hand (right).

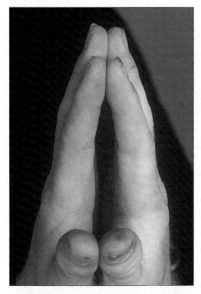

1.19 Joint stiffness in a long-standing diabetic. The 'prayer sign' is caused by irreversible glycosylation of tissue proteins.

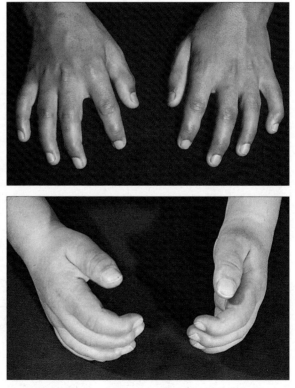

1.20, 1.21 Claw hands in two children with storage disorders (mucolipidosis 3 [top] and Hunter syndrome [bottom]).

short fingers (brachydactyly) in many syndromes associated with short stature (**1.26**). Only the fifth finger may be shortened, as in Coffin–Siris syndrome (**1.27**), or just one or two metacarpals as in pseudo-hypoparathyroidism (**1.28**, **1.29**). Fingers may show fusion (syndactyly), or duplication with or without fusion (polydactyly or polysyndactyly) (**1.30**, **1.31**), in some dysmorphic syndromes. All the fingers may be bent, as in various of the camptodactyly syndromes associated with short stature (**1.32**) or just the fifth finger (clinodactyly), which is a non-specific abnormality in many syndromic disorders (**1.33**). A myopathic or rheumatic hand may show ulnar drift (**1.34**). A trident hand is seen in achondroplasia (**1.35**). The thumb may be broad (**1.36**), triphalangeal (**1.37**) or low set (**1.38**) in various syndromes. The finger tips and interphalangeal joints are broad in Aarskog syndrome (**1.39**), a dominantly inherited condition associated with moderate short stature. The wrist is expanded in rickets for whatever cause (**1.40**). Clubbing is seen in chronic cyanotic heart disease, chronic purulent respiratory disorders and inflammatory bowel disease as well as occurring dominantly in families (**1.41**). The nails may be deep set in the Sotos syndrome of cerebral gigantism (**1.42**) and hypoplastic in those syndromes characterized by early lymphedema such as the Ullrich–Turner syndrome (**1.43**, **1.44**). The palms show a yellowish discoloration in true pituitary gigantism and hypothyroidism (**1.45**) or may show redness in chronic liver disorders. Now move up to inspect the arms.

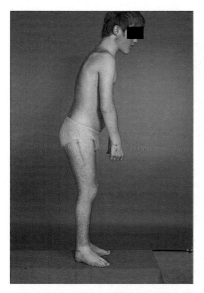

1.22 Generalized skin stiffness in a child producing limited joint mobility and short stature.

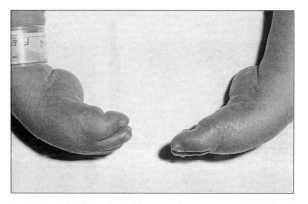

1.23 Fixed joint contractures or arthrogryposis, here presenting as bilateral talipes in a child with camptodactyly and prenatal onset short stature.

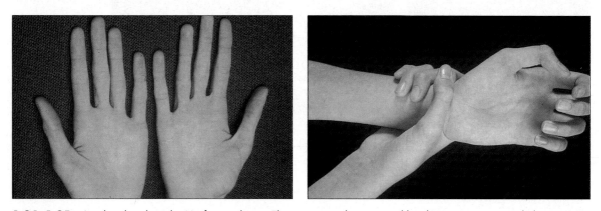

1.24, 1.25 Arachnodactyly in the Marfan syndrome. The wrist sign, demonstrated by clasping one wrist with the opposite hand and noting overlap of the distal phalanges of thumb and middle finger.

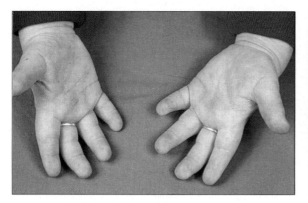

1.26 Brachydactyly. This is found in many syndromes associated with short stature.

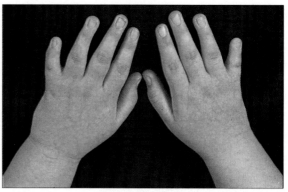

1.27 Short fifth digit in Coffin–Siris syndrome.

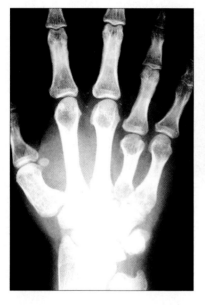

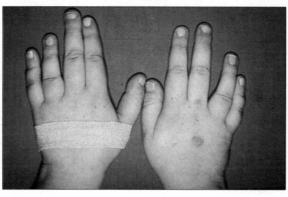

1.28, 1.29 Short fourth and fifth metacarpals seen in hand of child with pseudohypoparathyroidism.

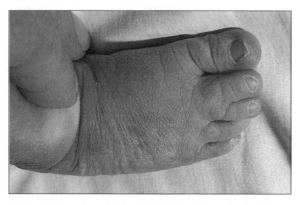

1.30 Syndactyly. A normal, often familial, variant and a non-specific clue to look for other dysmorphic features.

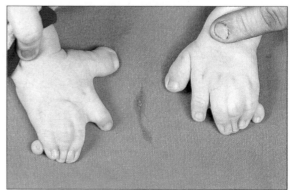

1.31 Polysyndactyly, here in the Carpenter syndrome.

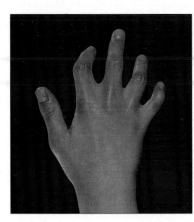

1.32 Camptodactyly. There is a group of camptodactyly syndromes associated with short stature and scoliosis.

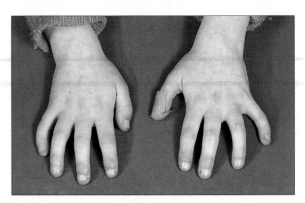

1.33 Clinodactyly. This is found in many syndromes associated with short stature.

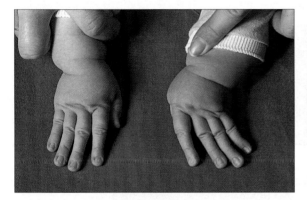

1.34 Myopathic hand in child with coexistent growth hormone deficiency and severe scoliosis.

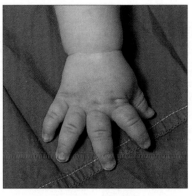

1.35 Trident hand in achondroplasia.

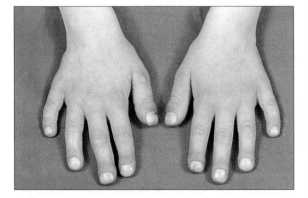

1.36 Broad thumb as seen in Rubinstein–Taybi syndrome.

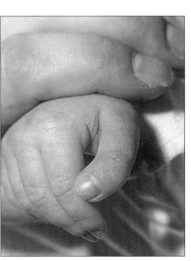

1.37 Triphalangeal thumb.

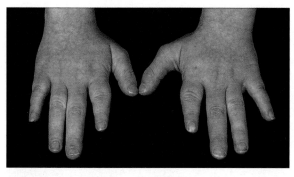

1.38 Low set thumb.

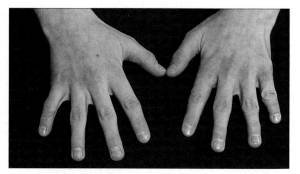

1.39 Expanded interphalangeal joints and finger tips in Aarskog syndrome.

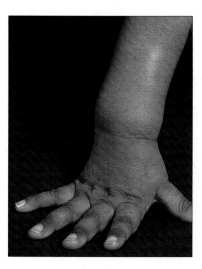

1.40 Expansion of the wrist in nutritional rickets.

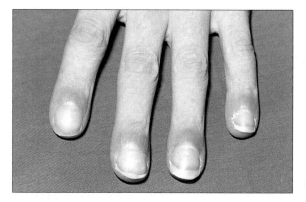

1.41 Clubbing, here in a case of cystic fibrosis.

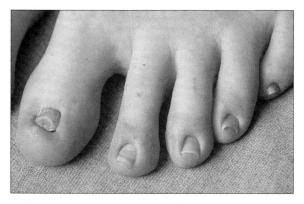

1.42 Deep-set nails in Sotos syndrome.

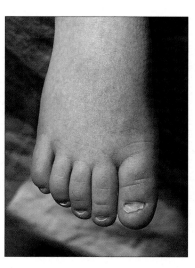

1.43 Hypoplastic nails as seen in around 40% of girls with the Ullrich–Turner syndrome.

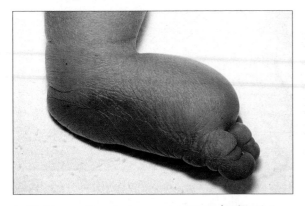

1.44 Neonatal lymphedema seen in 75% of girls with the Ullrich–Turner syndrome.

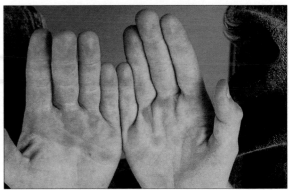

1.45 Yellow palmar discoloration in pituitary gigantism (also seen in hypothyroidism).

THE ARMS

The relative length of the arms can be assessed by measurement of span, as described above. Fixed flexion of the elbow and wrist may be seen with arthrogryposis and limited rotation of the forearm in some of the skeletal dysplasias (**1.40**). Radial aplasia or hypoplasia may be seen in some dysmorphic short stature syndromes and is associated with congenital heart defects, renal or hematological abnormalities (**1.47**). An increased carrying angle (**1.48**) is classically seen in the Ullrich–Turner syndrome (although it is absent in 50% of cases) and may be present in other syndromes.

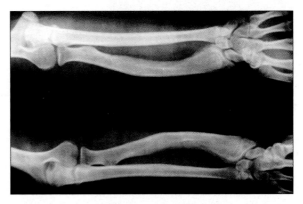

1.46 Radiograph of forearm in Leri-Weill dyschondrosteosis with bowed radius producing limited forearm rotation.

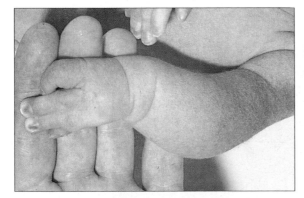

1.47 Radial hypoplasia in the Holt–Oram syndrome, associated with atrial and ventricular septal defects.

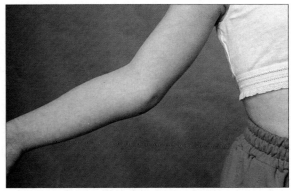

1.48 Increased carrying angle as seen in 50% of girls with Ullrich–Turner syndrome.

THE HEAD AND NECK

There are many abnormalities of this region that may indicate pathology and a selection of these are given in **1.49** through to **1.80**.

Redundant skin at the site of previous fetal nuchal edema is a feature of the Down, Ullrich–Turner and other chromosomal syndromes in the neonatal period (**1.49**, **1.50**) and may be more obvious than webbing at this stage. Webbing of the neck (**1.51**) is seen in 70% of cases of the Ullrich–Turner syndrome, although it is not a specific finding, and a short neck with a low hairline (**1.52–1.54**) is also seen in many dysmorphic syndromes. The shape of the face and

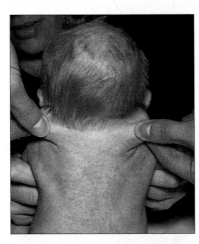

1.49 Loose skin of neck in neonate with the Down syndrome.

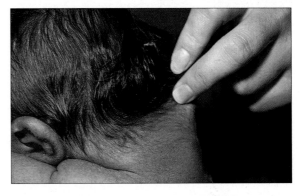

1.50 Loose skin of neck in neonate with the Ullrich–Turner syndrome.

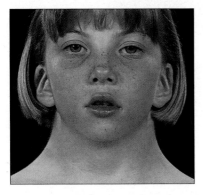

1.51 Later webbing of the neck in a case of the Noonan syndrome (as seen to some degree in 70% of girls with the Ullrich–Turner syndrome).

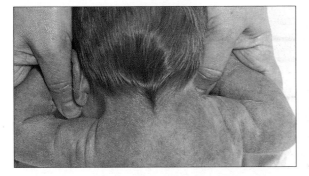

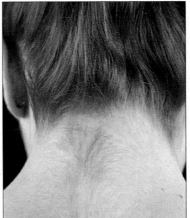

1.52, 1.53 Low hair line with mid-line extension seen in 75% of girls with Ullrich–Turner syndrome, shown in neonate (above) and late childhood (right).

skull (**1.55**), hypertelorism (**1.56**) or the presence of epicanthic folds, ptosis (**1.57**), ex- or enophthalmos (**1.58**, **1.59**) should be assessed along with the mouth and palate. Sub-mucous cleft palate may be revealed only by palpation. Any abnormalities of the mid-line are especially significant as they may indicate an associated abnormality of the pituitary gland (**1.60–1.63**). A high arched palate may be seen in the

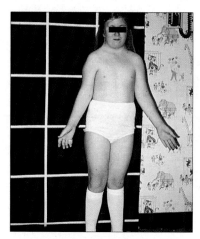

1.54 Short neck due to vertebral abnormalities (the Klippel–Feil malformation) producing an appearance superficially similar to the Ullrich–Turner syndrome.

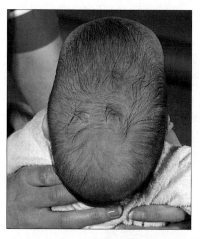

1.55 Dolichocephaly from craniosynostosis.

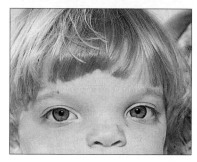

1.56 Severe hypertelorism.

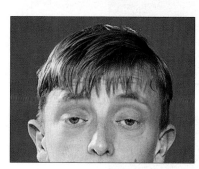

1.57 Ptosis as seen in 25% of girls with the Ullrich–Turner, the majority of children with the Noonan and more than 50 other dysmorphic syndromes.

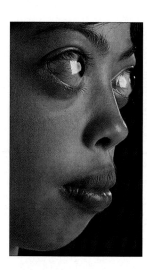

1.58 Exophthalmos in thyrotoxicosis.

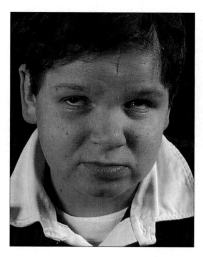

1.59 Enophthalmos in child with blindness and hypopituitarism secondary to basal astrocytoma.

Marfan, the Ullrich–Turner and some other dysmorphic syndromes (**1.64**).

The tongue is smooth (**1.65**) in iron deficiency for any cause and, in older age groups, in pernicious anemia where it may be associated with other autoimmune disease. Both the tongue and lips may show neuromata in neurofibromatosis (see below) and in the multiple endocrine adenomatosis type 2b syndrome

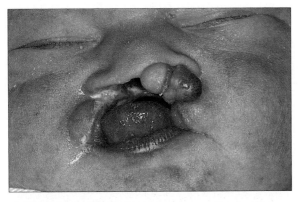

1.60 Cleft lip and palate, in this case associated with panhypopituitarism.

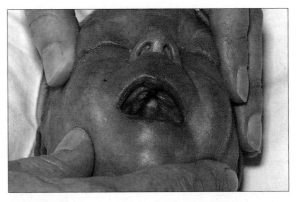

1.61 Cleft palate in Smith–Lemli–Opitz syndrome.

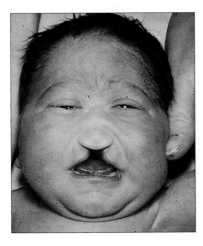

1.62 Mid line cleft and abnormal nose in holoprosencephaly. There may be associated panhypopituitarism.

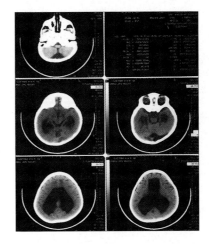

1.63 CT scan of same case demonstrating abnormal mid-line structures and clover-leaf ventricles.

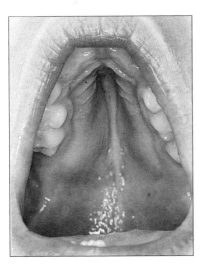

1.64 High arched palate seen in 75% of girls with Ullrich–Turner syndrome and the majority of cases of Marfan syndrome.

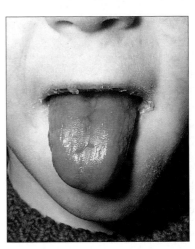

1.65 Smooth tongue in severe iron deficiency.

(**1.66**). The lips may be swollen and 'fish-like' in Crohn's disease (**1.67**). Oral candidiasis outside the neonatal period (**1.68**) may signal type 1 diabetes mellitus, immunodeficiency associated with hypoparathyroidism in DiGeorge syndrome and the autoimmune polyglandular type 1 or 'HAM' syndrome of Hypoparathyroidism, Adrenal failure and Moniliasis.

The teeth may be unusually soft and carious in disorders affecting collagen, fibrin and calcium metabolism and peg-like in ectodermal dysplasia (**1.69**). The teeth are an abnormal shape in the Rubinstein–Taybi syndrome (**1.70**). They may be stained or rotted by drugs and bilirubin (**1.71**). A single central incisor (**1.72**) is associated with congenital growth hormone

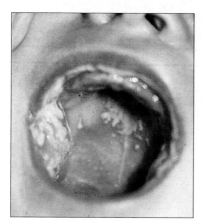

1.66 Glossal and labial neuromata in multiple endocrine adenomatosis type 2b.

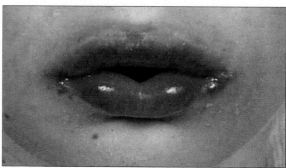

1.67 'Fish-lips' in oral Crohn's disease.

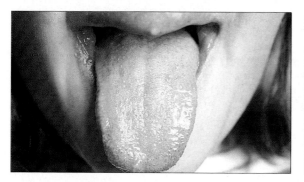

1.68 Oral candidiasis. If seen outside infancy then exclude diabetes mellitus, immunodeficiency and autoimmune disease.

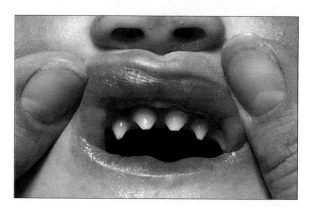

1.69 Peg-like teeth in ectodermal dysplasia.

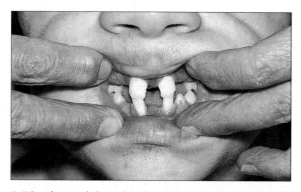

1.70 Abnormal shaped teeth in Rubinstein–Taybi syndrome.

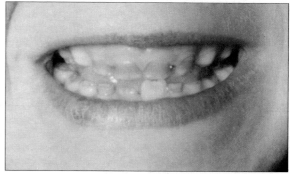

1.71 Bilirubin staining after severe jaundice in premature neonate with sustained growth failure.

deficiency. An assessment of the presence and number of the primary dentition and appearance of the secondary teeth can give clues to skeletal age and physiological maturity (see below). Delayed eruption of the teeth is seen in any disorder that delays physical maturation (especially chronic disease, hypothyroidism and hypopituitarism), in cleidocranial

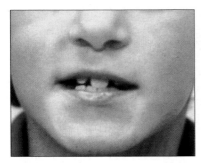

1.72 Single central incisor associated with congenital growth hormone deficiency.

dysostosis (**1.73**, **1.74**) and some other dysmorphic syndromes associated with short stature.

The ears are low set with or without rotation (**1.75**), or folded in an abnormal manner (**1.76**) in a host of dysmorphic syndromes associated with short stature.

Head hair may be abnormally sparse or curled in several syndromic and metabolic disorders and progeria (**1.77–1.79**). It may show abnormal patterns of whorl formation with underlying CNS malformation. Alopecia may indicate autoimmune disease and temporal hair loss is a feature of hypothyroidism (**1.80**).

Palpation of the neck, from behind the patient, will allow assessment of the size and shape of the thyroid gland, which should also be measured at its widest point across the isthmus and from top to base on both sides of the mid-line. Most goiters in childhood (see Chapter 7) are smooth, although nodular enlargement may rarely occur. They move upwards on swallowing and it is useful to have a glass of water at hand for this purpose. Aberrant lingual thyroid tissue may be visible in the mouth at the root of the tongue on swallowing. Retrosternal thyroid tissue can be identified by ultrasonography or lateral radiograph of the thoracic inlet.

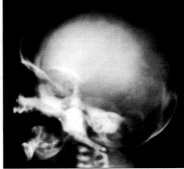

1.73, 1.74 Extreme delay of dental eruption is seen in cleidocranial dysostosis. (Hypothyroidism may produce similar gross delay.)

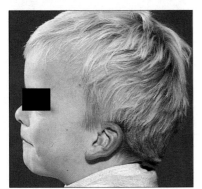

1.75 Low set, backward rotated ears.

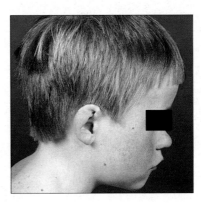

1.76 Abnormal helical pattern in pseudohypoparathyroidism.

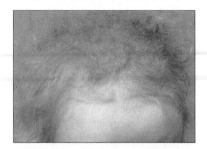

1.77 Sparse head hair in Russell–Silver syndrome.

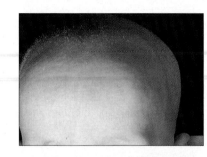

1.78 Menkes' kinky wool hair syndrome, a disorder of copper metabolism associated with prenatal onset short stature.

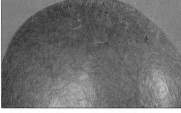

1.79 Hair-loss in progeria.

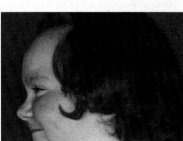

1.80 Temporal thinning of the hair in female with gross hypothyroidism.

THE CHEST, ABDOMEN AND CARDIOVASCULAR SYSTEM

These main systems should be examined to exclude any organic disorders that could produce poor growth or mimic an endocrinopathy. It is especially important to measure the blood pressure, as hypertension may be a feature of pheochromocytoma, CNS tumors, neurofibromatosis, the Cushing and Conn syndromes, ovarian tumors and some disorders of adrenal steroid biosynthesis. Hypertension in the right arm is also a feature of coarctation of the aorta which may be present in 40% of girls with Ullrich–Turner syndrome, and so the femoral pulses must also be assessed.

Major heart malformations and abnormal chest shape, such as pectus excavatum or pectus carinatum (**1.81, 1.82**), may be seen in many syndromes associated with both short and tall stature. A rachitic rosary may be seen (**1.83**). Many of the storage disorders, syndromic malformations and disorders of bone and collagen metabolism may show a scoliosis or kyphoscoliosis (**1.84**). The degree of angulation of the spine can be assessed radiographically (**1.85**) or by surface mapping techniques (**1.86**), and the loss of height quantified by measurement of sitting height.

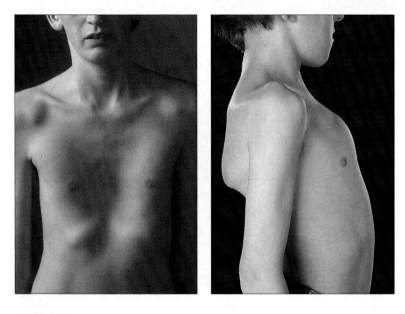

1.81, 1.82 Pectus excavatum in Marfan's syndrome. Pectus carinatum in the Noonan syndrome.

There may be abdominal organomegaly in some of the storage disorders, thalassemia and Beckwith–Wiedemann syndrome, where an umbilical hernia or omphalocele can also be seen (**1.87**). Inspection of the anal margin may reveal signs of sexual abuse or chronic inflammatory bowel disease (**1.88**).

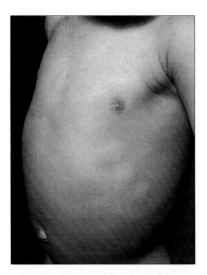

1.83 A rachitic rosary in a case of cystinosis.

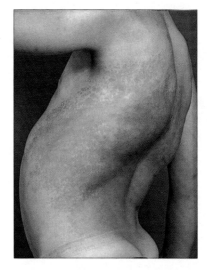

1.84 Scoliosis with plexiform neuroma in neurofibromatosis.

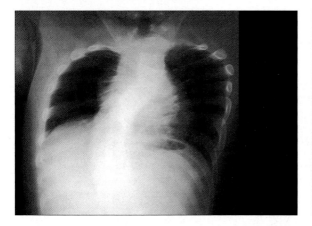

1.85 Radiograph of scoliosis in camptodactyly syndrome of the Tel–Hashomer variety.

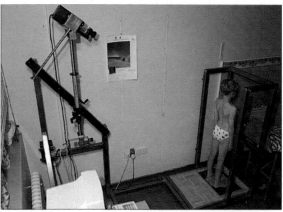

1.86 Assessing scoliosis using laser surface mapping.

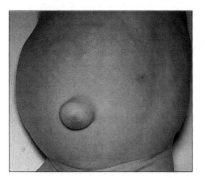

1.87 Umbilical hernia and visible organomegaly in Beckwith–Wiedemann syndrome.

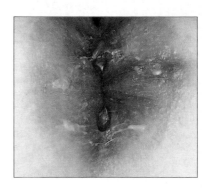

1.88 Anal signs of Crohn's disease.

THE BREASTS

Breast tissue and the pectoralis major muscle may be absent congenitally in the Poland sequence (**1.89**). (There may also be associated heart defects.) It may be damaged or destroyed after bilateral neonatal breast abscesses (**1.90**), or after misguided surgery for abscess or physiological neonatal gynecomastia (**1.91**). Physiological gynecomastia in the adolescent male is common and may be seen especially in the obese individual (**1.92**), possibly requiring surgical resection. Pathological causes of early breast development will be discussed in Chapter 4. Virginal breast hypertrophy (juvenile fibroadenoma) is uncommon but dramatic (**1.93**). Accessory nipples are common (**1.94**) and it is rare, but possible, for them to overlie significant breast tissue. Gentle pressure may demonsrate infected or milky discharge.

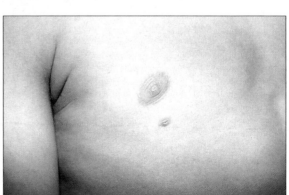

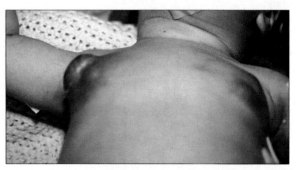

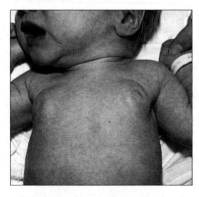

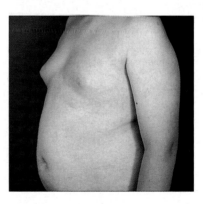

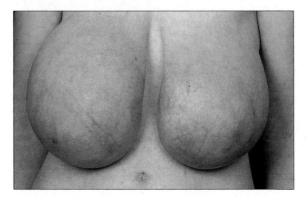

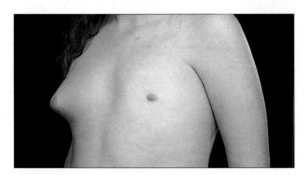

1.89 Poland sequence. There is absence of the left pectoralis major and breast tissue. This child was referred with unilateral breast enlargement – a good example of normal stage 4 breast development.

1.90 Neonatal breast abscess. Delayed antibiotic therapy or mistaken surgical intervention can lead to later amastia.

1.91 Physiological neonatal gynecomastia.

1.92 Male gynecomastia with moderate obesity.

1.93 Virginal breast hypertrophy (juvenile fibroadenoma).

1.94 Accessory nipple.

THE GENITALIA

Many endocrine disorders have associated abnormalities of the genitalia and these will be dealt with in detail in Chapters 4, 5 and 6.

Look especially in both sexes for signs of herniae (or the scars of their repair early in life). In all patients presenting with a possible endocrine disorder a full assessment of physical maturity is mandatory. It is usual to stage the appearance of the pubic hair, penis and testicular volume in the male and the appearance of the breast, pubic hair and the onset of menstrua-tion in a girl. Details of this staging are given in **1.95** and illustrated in **1.96–1.99.** Menarche is recorded as an all-or-nothing event (although regular periods may take time to establish). Testicular volume is record-ed directly by comparison to an orchidometer (**1.98**). The onset of puberty (≥4 ml testes) is followed by the onset of the pubertal growth spurt after about 6 months. Peak height velocity is attained with 12–14 ml testicular volume. Other secondary sexual char-acteristics should be noted, such as acne (**1.100**), axillary hair, vaginal discharge and an adult body odor. In an individual, any discrepancy between the

Stages of sexual maturation and mean growth potential

Male and female pubic hair

Stage	Male	Female
1	None	None
2	Barely visible at base of penis or on scrotum	Barely visible on mons or labia
3	More visible, same sites as stage 2	More visible, same sites as stage 2
4	More extensive and dark; extending to suprapubic region	More extensive and dark; extending to suprapubic region
5	Adult triangle with extension onto medial aspects of thighs	Adult triangle
5+	Extension upwards in midline	Extension upwards in midline and onto medial aspects of thighs

Male genital stages

Stage	
1	Prepubertal penis
2	Beginning of enlargement, more in length than breadth; scrotal skin thickens
3	Further enlargement and early separation of contour of glans from shaft
4	Near adult shape, not fully grown; scrotal skin dark and thick
5	Adult penis

Female breast stages

Stage	
1	Prepubertal
2	Breast bud palpable (onset of pubertal height spurt)
3	Obvious elevation of breast tissue (PHV)
4	Areola and nipple separate on enlarging breast*
5	Adult size and shape; areola and nipple merge

* Some normal girls will not pass this stage.

Mean growth potential for different stages of puberty, (range) in centimeters

Stage	Male		Female	
2-PHV	12.5	(2.9–28.7)	6.8	(0–16.3)
2-final	27.9	(17.9–41.2)	21.0	(11.6–29.4)
3-final	20.3	(3.9–30.1)	13.7	(6.1–21.6)
PHV-final	5.7	(9.6–22.6)	14.4	(8.6–23.0)
4-final	14.6	(1.1–25.2)	7.5	(2.7–13.7)
5-final	8.4	(0–20.5)	3.8	(0–10.0)
Menarche-final	–		5.8	(1–12.7)

Data courtesy of Dr JM Buckler

1.95 Stages of sexual maturation and growth potential. PHV = peak height velocity.

stages of sexual development is of particular importance (**1.101**) (see Chapter 4).

Shawl scrotum (**1.102**), where the root of the penis lies within the upper scrotum, and which is often bifid (**1.103**), is seen in several dysmorphic syndromes, especially the Aarskog syndrome. Other apparently minor abnormalities of genital architecture may have significance in the context of other physical findings.

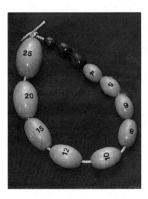

1.96 Female pubic hair stages 1-5+.

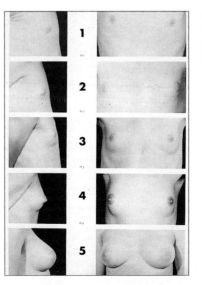

1.97 Male penis and pubic hair development stages 1–5+.

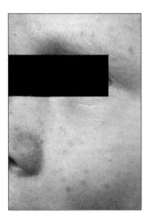

1.98 Prader orchidometer graded from 1 ml to 25 ml. The achievement of pubertal 4 ml testes is shown by a change from blue to yellow beads.

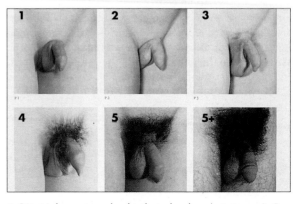

1.99 Female breast development stages 1–5.

1.100 Early acne in 6 year old with adrenal hyperplasia.

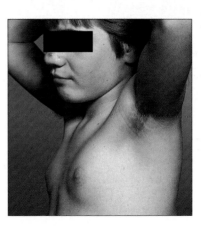

1.101 Excess adrenal steroids. Acne and axillary hair are excessive for the stage of breast development.

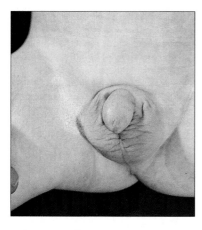

1.102 Shawl scrotum.

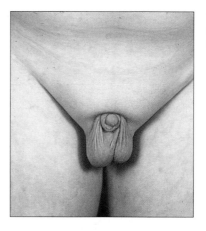

1.103 Bifid scrotum. (See also chapter 6.)

SKELETAL MATURITY

Although not strictly part of the examination of a child, it is pertinent to discuss here a complementary, radiographic, means of establishing physiological maturity. The most commonly used methods involve assessing the number and degree of development of the bones of the left hand and wrist (**1.104**), although other growth centers can be used including the jaw and teeth. Several methods exist for scoring or 'aging' the individual ossification centers in comparison to a standard atlas or using a computer recognition system. It is then possible, by using published equations incorporating current height, or in some cases height and recent height velocity, to calculate a predicted adult height (with a range of error of ± 2 SD).

THE CENTRAL NERVOUS SYSTEM AND EYES

Examination here should concentrate on an assessment of developmental or educational level and an exclusion of major neurological abnormality. It is particularly important to examine the optic discs that might demonstrate papilledema (**1.105**) secondary to raised intracranial pressure. The pallor of optic atrophy (**1.106**) may be secondary to compression by a local tumor or raised intracranial pressure, or found in the DIDMOAD syndrome (Diabetes Insipidus, Diabetes Mellitus, Optic Atrophy and Deafness). The visual fields (**1.107**, **1.108**) may show bitemporal restriction in the presence of compression of the optic chiasm by a craniopharyngioma. The retina may be dysplastic with small optic nerve heads in

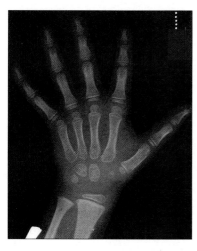

1.104 Left wrist and hand radiograph for bone age estimation.

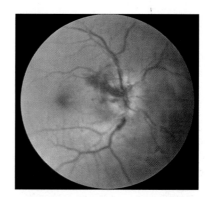

1.105 Papilledema in craniopharyngioma, placed posteriorly to the pituitary and causing secondary hydrocephalus.

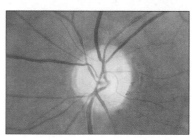

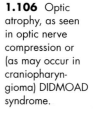

1.106 Optic atrophy, as seen in optic nerve compression or (as may occur in craniopharyngioma) DIDMOAD syndrome.

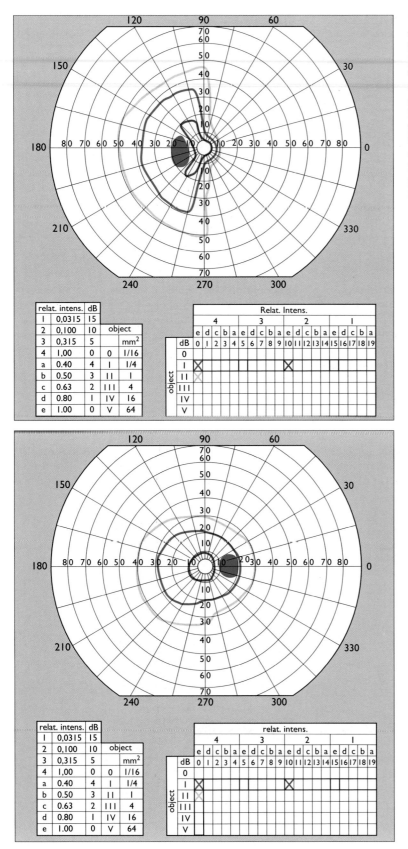

1.107, 1.108 Visual fields in a child with craniopharyngioma. There is temporal hemianopia in the left eye (**1.107**) and generalized restriction of vision in the right eye (**1.108**) secondary to compression of the optic chiasm. This formal plotting is possible in older, co-operative children. In the young child, the presence of temporal field loss can be demonstrated by confrontation or by bringing a small, interesting object inwards from the periphery, close to the child's face and noting when there is a reaction.

septo-optic dysplasia (**1.109**, **1.110**) associated with panhypopituitarism or isolated pituitary hormone deficiencies with or without mid-line brain abnormalities. Retinitis pigmentosa (**1.111**) is seen in several syndromes associated with short stature, for instance the Laurence–Moon syndrome (with obesity, spasticity, learning difficulties and hypogonadism), or the similar Bardet–Biedl syndrome (with obesity, polydactyly, learning difficulties and hypogonadism). Storage deposits may be visible either in the retinae (**1.112**) or lens. The lens shows dislocation or loose fixation, said to be more commonly upwards in the Marfan syndrome and more commonly downwards in homocystinuria (**1.113**).

The eyes might show abnormal blue coloration of the cornea in disorders of collagen metabolism (**1.114**). A nevus of Ota can be associated with intracranial hamartomas and sexual precocity (**1.115**). There may be abnormal sparsity, duplication or luxuriance of the eyelashes in several syndromes associated with short stature (**1.116**).

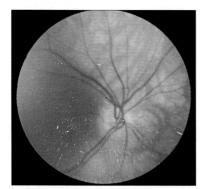

1.109 Retinal dysplasia in septo-optic dysplasia (de Morsier syndrome).

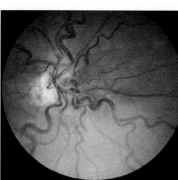

1.110 Absent mid-line structures in same patient as **1.109**.

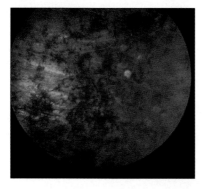

1.111 Retinitis pigmentosa in the Laurence—Moon syndrome.

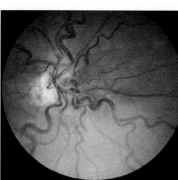

1.112 Pseudopapilledema caused by abnormal storage deposits in geleophysic dwarfism.

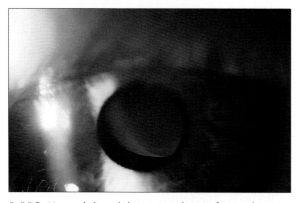

1.113 Upwards lens dislocation in the Marfan syndrome.

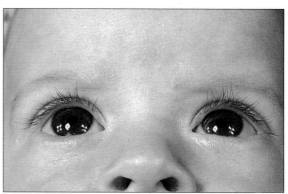

1.114 Blue sclerae in the commonest, Type 1, osteogenesis imperfecta.

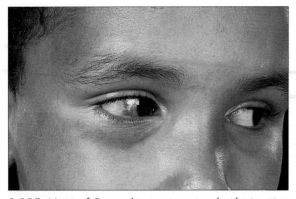

1.115 Nevus of Ota, in this case associated with gigantism and sexual precocity due to hypothalamic dysfunction.

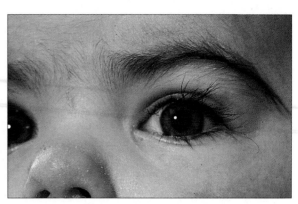

1.116 Long eyelashes in De Lange syndrome.

BODY SHAPE AND THE SKIN

Look at the general shape of the body and at the distribution of muscle and fat. Abnormal muscularity may be seen in non-salt losing males with the adrenogenital syndrome and in anabolic steroid abuse in young adolescents. Generalized lipodystrophy is seen in progeria and in the 'leprechaun' and related syndromes where there may be associated insulin resistance (**1.117**). Localized lipoatrophy is seen in relation to injection sites of porcine insulin (**1.118**) and in some specific lipoatrophy syndromes. Local lipohypertrophy is seen in relation to human insulin and growth hormone (**1.119**). Excess adiposity is a feature of many endocrine disorders and may show a peculiar dimpled appearance in hypopituitarism (**1.120**).

Hemihypertrophy may affect the whole body (**1.121**) or isolated areas such as one side of the face or one limb (**1.122**). Asymmetry is associated with Russell–Silver dwarfism, Beckwith–Wiedemann syndrome and, in the isolated form, may also increase the risk of Wilms' tumor. Local hypertrophy of a limb in association with hemangiomata (Klippel–Trenaunay–Weber syndrome) may also occur (**1.123**) (see Chapter 3).

Neurofibromatosis (see Chapters 2 and 4) is signaled by neuromas (**1.124**) or a large number of café au lait spots (**1.125**), which may be discrete or large and plexiform (**1.126**), and axillary freckling. The edge of these spots is said to be relatively smooth like the coastline of California. The café au lait spot in McCune–Albright syndrome (**1.127**) associated with sexual precocity (see Chapter 4) has a rough outline like the coast of Maine. Multiple pigmented nevi (**1.128**) are associated with a number of syndromic malformations and neuroectodermal tumors.

Skin pigmentation may be abnormally increased with over secretion of ACTH as in Addisonism and

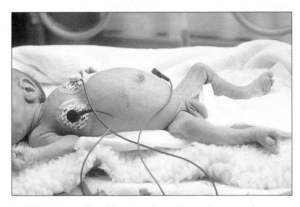

1.117 Generalized lipoatrophy in Leprechaun syndrome.

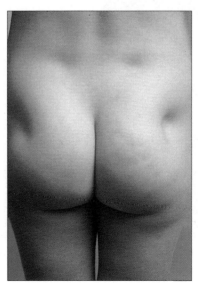

1.118 Lipoatrophy at animal insulin injection sites.

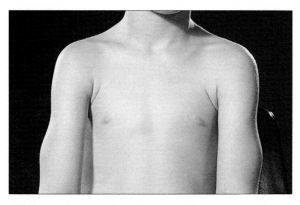

1.120 Abnormal abdominal fat in hypopituitarism.

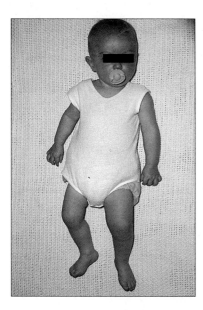

1.119 Lipohypertrophy at human insulin injection sites.

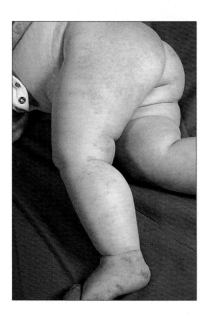

1.121 Generalized left sided hemihypertrophy.

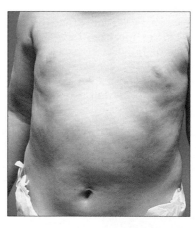

1.122 Isolated hemihypertrophy of right leg.

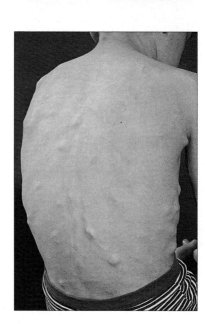

1.123 Overgrowth of limb in Klippel—Trenaunay—Weber syndrome with cavernous hemangioma.

1.124 Multiple neuromas in neurofibromatosis.

Nelson syndrome (see Chapters 2 and 8) and this may be generalized (**1.129**) or localized to scar tissue (**1.130**). Coal black discoloration of the axillae or neck (acanthosis nigricans) (**1.131, 1.132**) is associated with insulin resistance and obesity. Vitiligo (**1.133**) is commonly an isolated disorder but may be associ-ated with several of the polyglandular syndromes (see Chapter 8).

Easy bruising and skin fragility is seen in the tissue paper scarring of Ehlers–Danlos syndrome (**1.134**); skin laxity is also increased (**1.135**). Non-accidental bruising and burns indicate physical abuse (**1.136, 1.137**).

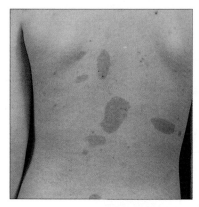

1.125 Café au lait spots in neurofibromatosis. Note the relatively smooth outline.

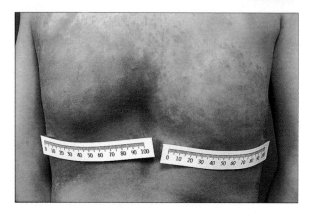

1.126 Plexiform neuroma in neurofibromatosis.

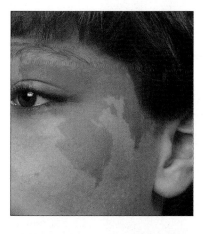

1.127 Café au lait spot in McCune–Albright syndrome. Note irregular border.

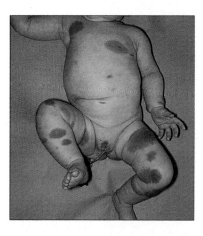

1.128 Multiple pigmented nevi, here associated with later intracranial malignant change at 3 years of age.

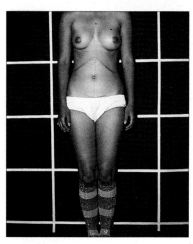

1.129 Generalized hyperpigmentation in Nelson's syndrome.

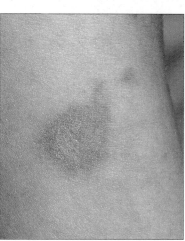

1.130 Scar pigmentation in Addisonism.

The Cushing syndrome in childhood is often associated with easy bruising. A particular feature of childhood onset Cushing syndrome is marked hirsutism, which is also a feature of other disorders of the adrenal gland and ovary characterized by overproduction of testosterone (see Chapters 3, 4 and 8). Hirsutism is also seen as part of the fetal alcohol syndrome (see below). Treatment with some drugs, such as metyrapone, can also cause hirsutism. The use of diazoxide in hyperinsulinism causes generalized and non-pigmented hypertrichosis (**1.138**). Retention of excess lanugo hair may

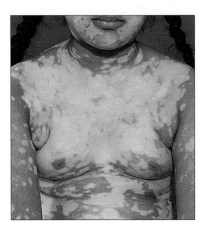

1.131 Axillary acanthosis nigricans

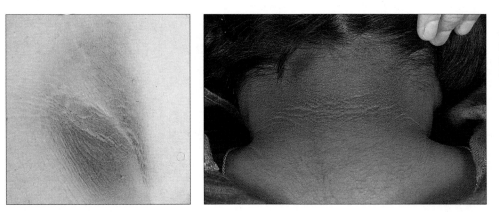

1.132 The same condition affecting the neck in Asian patient with insulin resistance.

1.133 Severe vitiligo in polyglandular syndrome type 1.

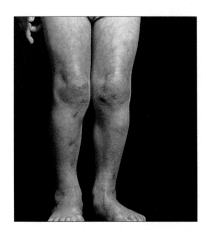

1.134 Tissue paper scars from excess skin fragility in Ehlers–Danlos syndrome.

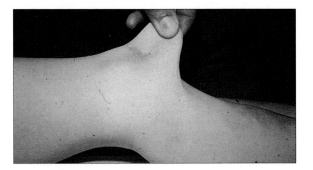

1.135 Extensible skin in Ehlers–Danlos syndrome

be seen in Aarskog syndrome (**1.139**) and in anorexia nervosa. Striae are a feature especially of iatrogenic Cushing syndrome (**1.140**) and may be also seen in nutritional obesity and in tall stature (see Chapter 3).

Dry skin is seen in atopic disorders, ectodermal dysplasia, and may be also atrophic, as in progeria (**1.141**) and some other dysmorphic syndromes. Excessive lichenification is seen in the X-linked metabolic disorder, placental sulfatase deficiency (**1.142**), when the affected

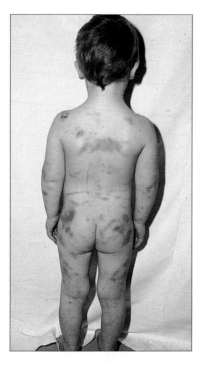

1.136 Child abuse. Multiple bruises. Note the characteristic shortened lower body segment which may mimic hypochondroplasia.

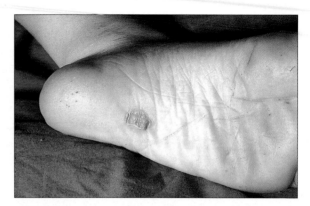

1.137 Child abuse. Cigarette burn to soles of feet.

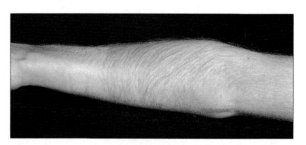

1.139 Downy body hair in Aarskog syndrome

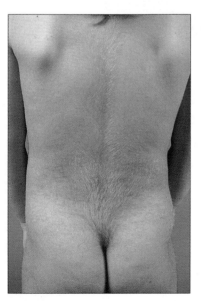

1.138 Hypertrichosis secondary to diazoxide treatment. Also seen with cyclosporin.

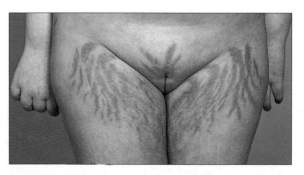

1.140 Striae in iatrogenic Cushing syndrome.

fetus will be post-mature and maternal estriol levels will have been undetectable during pregnancy. Dry, fissured reddening of the palms and soles is seen in 3A syndrome of adrenal failure, alacrima and achalasia, progressive nervous system degeneration may also occur (**1.143**).

Necrobiosis lipoidica and granuloma annulare have associations with insulin dependent diabetes mellitus (**1.144**, **1.145**). Dimpling of the skin is seen in hypophosphatasia where there is under-mineralization of the skeleton and teeth and, in the childhood form, short stature (**1.146**).

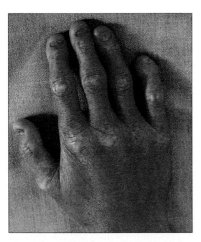

1.141 Atrophic skin on hands in progeria.

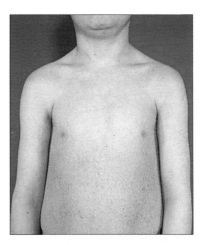

1.142 Lichenification of skin in placental sulfatase deficiency.

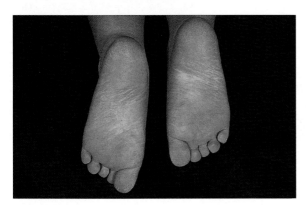

1.143 Red fissured feet in the 3A syndrome.

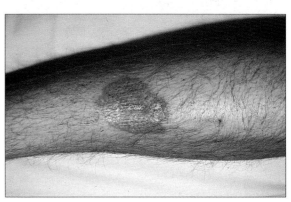

1.144 Necrobiosis lipoidica in insulin dependent diabetes mellitus (IDDM).

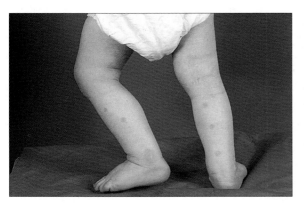

1.145 Granuloma annulare in IDDM.

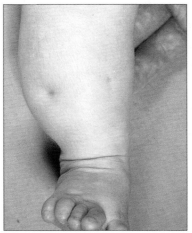

1.146 Dimpling over tibia in hypophospha-tasia.

THE PARENTS

If at all possible, it is important to examine the parents briefly. They may provide valuable clues as to the diagnosis. Many skeletal dysplasias and some dysmorphic syndromes associated with both tall and short stature are dominantly inherited and may be more obvious in later life. A parent, more often the mother, may show signs of undiagnosed hypo- or hyperthyroidism and the mother may be mildly affected by a metabolic disorder, such as phenylketonuria or myotonic dystrophy, that has severely affected the infant (**1.147**). A wide philtrum and a thin upper lip may be seen in the offspring of heavy drinkers during pregnancy, along with short stature, learning difficulties, hirsutism and limb abnormalities (**1.148**).

The cardinal features to include in the examination of a child with a possible growth or endocrine disorder are summarized in the table (**1.149**).

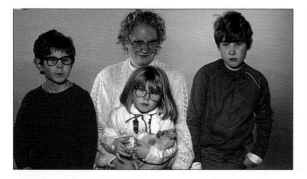

1.147 Undiagnosed mild maternal phenylketonuria affecting offspring. All the children are short. The female child has severe learning difficulties. Mother has fair hair and blue eyes.

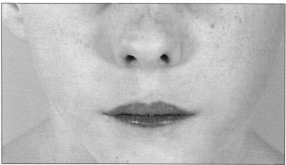

1.148 Fetal alcohol syndrome in later childhood showing typical facies.

1.149 Essential points on physical examination.

Essential points on physical examination

Auxology (including parents) and bone age
Any abnormalities of the hands / feet, nails or arms?
Any abnormalities of the head and neck (with special reference to the midline, mouth, tongue and thyroid)?
Any chest wall (including breast) or spine abnormalities?
Any cardiovascular or respiratory abnormalities?
Any abdominal abnormalities (must include external genital inspection)?
Stage of sexual maturation
Any abnormal skin or fat signs?
Any abnormal body shape or asymmetry?
Any eye abnormalities including lens, visual fields and retinae?
Is there an abnormal appearance of either of the parents?

2.

The Short Child

PHYSIOLOGY

Human growth hormone (hGH) is a single-chain 191 amino acid polypeptide that circulates complexed to a binding protein (see below), or is unbound ('free'). Multiple molecular forms of GH with various biological activities arise from post-translational processing. At all ages – fetal through adult – GH is secreted in an intermittent, pulsatile pattern largely due to the reciprocal interactions of two hypothalamic peptides, GH releasing hormone (GHRH) and somatostatin or GH release inhibiting factor (SRIF). As well as growth hormone itself there are a number of peptides (e.g. IGF-1) and neurotransmitters that control GH release. During childhood there are apparently no differences between the sexes, although several investigators have noted significant correlations between height or height velocity and the amount of GH secreted throughout the day.

Growth hormone interacts with its receptor to generate insulin-like growth factor-I (IGF-1), the main mediator of GH action, in the liver and at the epiphyses. This receptor, the extracellular domain of which is identical with the circulating GH binding protein, must link up with a second receptor molecule through a two site growth hormone bridge. This two receptor, one hGH molecular complex permits IGF-1 generation. In addition, GH circulating half-life is virtually doubled by the presence of the binding protein.

Many of the effects of GH are mediated by IGF-1 which circulates in the plasma bound to one of a series of binding proteins called IGFBPs. These proteins circulate and modify IGF-1 action – either as stimulators or inhibitors. Although there are at least six of the compounds, IGFBP-3 is the major circulating form.

This complex system subserves the process of growth. At puberty the pulsatile release of GH is increased 2 to 3 fold, predominantly by increased amounts of GH released at each secretory episode. Along with increasing amounts of sex steroid hormones this accounts for the majority of the pubertal growth spurt, following which the secretion of GH returns toward prepubertal values. Since the levels of the GH binding protein do not increase as much as GH secretion, there is an apparent imbalance between the amounts of GH and its binding protein permitting more GH to circulate in the active ('free') form. Theoretically, this increase also drives the local (e.g. epiphyseal) production of IGF-1 and its binding proteins and directly augments long bone growth.

Secretion of GH may be mediated by input from higher centers allowing for modification of growth rate by environmental and emotional factors. The process of growth is also dependent on adequate nutrition, normal bone structure and biochemistry, normal thyroxine and other endocrine secretion as well as general health. Disruption of normal growth may therefore be an indication of many pathologies. Genetic size is determined by inheritance from the parents, but the mechanisms underlying this programing of stature are obscure.

AETIOLOGY

There are many classifications of short stature, all with their advantages and disadvantages. None is perfect, as any group of disorders can be viewed as a spectrum in which dividing lines are often difficult to establish.

In this Chapter the classification is based on a separation between idiopathic, primary and secondary growth failure. This subdivision makes sense as growth failure can be caused either by an intrinsic disorder in the cells or structure of the growth plates (primary) or by an external influence on the growth plate (secondary). The first category, in which the mechanisms behind the short stature are purely familial, or unknown, is the commonest.

IDIOPATHIC SHORT STATURE

Idiopathic short stature is defined by the absence of abnormalities in the history and physical examination. More specifically, birth weight and length are normal, as well as body proportions; there is no chronic ill health, no severe psychosocial disturbance, and a normal food intake.

If growth velocity is normal, there is no need to exclude growth hormone deficiency or other pathologies by formal testing. If the growth curve deviates clearly, for example more than 0.3 standard deviations (SD) over 1 year or more than 0.5 SD over 2 years or if the calculated height velocity is below the 25th centile twice in a row, (with an adequate measurement interval), then a GH provocation test or a measurement of serum insulin-like growth factor-1 (IGF-1) and its binding protein (IGFBP-3) is undertaken, along with the screening tests described below. Idiopathic short stature can be sub-classified into 4 groups:

1. **Familial short stature** characterized by:
   - short stature during the growth period and a reduced final height compared to the normal mean.
   - a normal height velocity (varying around the 25th centile)*.
   - a height within the target range defined by parental size.
   - bone age consistent with chronological age (within 2 SD).
   - a normal age of onset of puberty.

As the height centile lines diverge with increasing age a short child on the 3rd height centile will show a velocity that varies around the 25th velocity centile. Similarly a tall child on the 97th centile will show variation around the 75th centile. The majority of children with 'normal' stature and an adequate gap between measurements will have a velocity that fluctuates within these limits.

2. **Constitutional delay of growth and adolescence** (CDGA) characterized by:
   - short stature during childhood.
   - stature below the range defined by parental size.
   - a retarded bone age (>2 SD below chronological age).
   - a reduced height velocity (<25%) in the later childhood years.
   - delayed onset of puberty.

Adult height is generally in the normal range. Often there is a positive family history of delayed puberty in the same sex parent. Strictly speaking, this diagnosis can be made only after the normal but late onset of puberty. However, the combination of the first four criteria strongly suggests this diagnosis, (see Chapter 5). The condition presents much more commonly in boys.

3. **A combination of both conditions** is often seen, and in fact the division between familial short stature and constitutional delay of growth and adolescence is to an extent artificial (**2.1**). Children with this combined form frequently present for medical assessment at a relatively young age, and, as height can be markedly reduced in adolescence, this can give rise to much concern.

4. **Unclassified**, if there are no positive arguments to classify the child in one of the above three groups, in the absence of a known cause. Mistaken or concealed paternity may be present in some cases.

PRIMARY GROWTH FAILURE

Five groups of disorders are found in this broad category.

1. Clinically defined syndromes with chromosomal abnormalities

These include the Ullrich–Turner syndrome (see also Chapter 5) and the Down syndrome. As the Ullrich––Turner syndrome is relatively common (1/2500 female births) and one of the few chromosomal or syndromic (see below) conditions in which the height deficit is potentially remediable, this will be described in detail.

The majority of Ullrich–Turner syndrome fetuses do not survive to term, but chromosomal analysis is not routinely performed on all miscarriages. The exact chromosomal make-up is very variable with just over half being due to the classical 45X karyotype and the remainder a variety of mosaics, chromosomal deletions and rings. Whatever the karyotype the phenotypic features are similar (including a reduced final height potential (see below), although the chances of spontaneous puberty may be greater in the mosaic forms.

Nuchal edema (also present in the Down syndrome) may be seen on second trimester ultrasound scanning and lead to diagnosis on amniocentesis.

Neonatal lymphedema (**2.2**) and the related nail dysplasia (**1.43**) may allow for an early diagnosis which should be suspected in all females with coarctation of the aorta (**2.3**). The major features of the condition are given in **2.4** and **2.7**, but it is important to note that up to 40% of girls will show no external features apart from reduced height (**2.5, 2.6**). Thus the diagnosis must be suspected in any girl presenting with short stature.

Final height in the condition is reduced to a mean of around 145–147 cm (depending on the population), but is related to parental height centile in the same way as a normal child. There are published centile charts for the condition and so a predicted final height may be obtained as described in Chapter 1 using the centile of both parents plotted on the final centile position of the Ullrich–Turner centiles.

2. Clinically defined syndromes without currently known chromosomal abnormalities

There are literally thousands of syndromes associated with short stature. Some of the features that may point to one of this multitude are given in Chapter 1.

An exact description of the majority of these disorders is beyond the scope of this text, but the reader may be aided by some of the commercially available computerized diagnostic databases or texts cited in the Suggested Reference Texts on page 143.

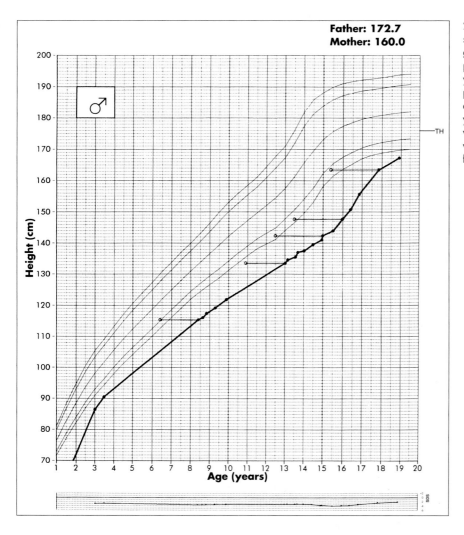

Father: 172.7
Mother: 160.0

2.1 Combined familial short stature and delay of growth and puberty. Both parents are short but the 3 year delay in the onset of puberty produces a fall from a height of -2 SDS at 14 years to -4 SDS at 16 years, with eventual recovery to within the genetic range for final height.

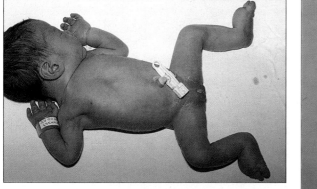

2.2 Neonatal lymphedema in Ullrich–Turner syndrome.

2.3 Shield-like chest and scar of coarctation repair in Ullrich–Turner syndrome.

Features of, and dissimilarities between, the Noonan and Ullrich–Turner syndromes

	Noonan	Ullrich–Turner
Sex	Either	Female
Chromosomes	Normal Dominant inheritance	45X, mosaic or abnormal X chromosome
Performance	Mild reduction in about 20%	Normal, some isolated performance deficits
Mean final height	Male 162 cm Female 152 cm	146 cm
Heart	Right sided abnormalities (80%) and cardiomyopathy (10–20%)	Left sided abnormalities including coarctation
Gonads	Males cryptorchid, Females normal	Streak ovaries
Eyes	Ptosis (majority)	Ptosis (minority)
Other	Café au lait spots Abnormal bleeding (70%)	Renal abnormalities

2.4 Features of, and dissimilarities between, the Noonan and Ullrich–Turner syndromes.

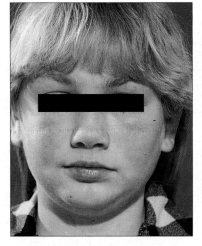

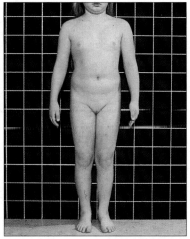

2.5, 2.6 Ullrich–Turner syndrome. Normal face and body phenotype (slightly broad chest).

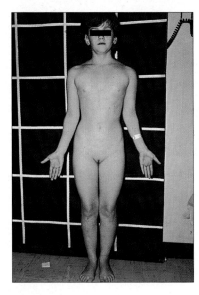

2.7 Broad chest, wide carrying angle and sexual infantilism in Ullrich–Turner syndrome age 15.5 years.

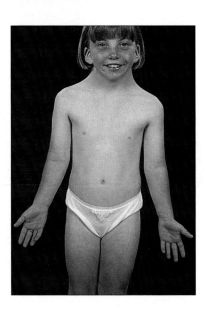

2.8 Noonan syndrome.

Among the most common and most important of syndromes presenting primarily with short stature are the Noonan (**2.8**), and Prader–Labhart–Willi (**2.9**, **2.10**). Noonan syndrome is common, with an incidence of approximately 1/2000 individuals. It is dominantly inherited with variable expression and there is some evidence from a large Dutch kindred that it maps to chromosome 12q. The Noonan syndrome shares many phenotypic features with the Ullrich–Turner syndrome; these are compared in 2.4. There is an overlap of some cases of the Noonan syndrome and neurofibromatosis, with some children showing multiple café au lait spots. The main features of Prader–Labhart–Willi syndrome are given in **2.11**.

Some syndromes have no known cause, normal intelligence and only relatively mild dysmorphic features and yet can produce the most striking degrees of short stature, an example of which, geleophysic dwarfism, is given (**2.12**, **2.13**).

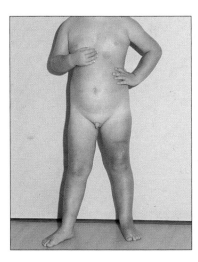

2.9 Prader–Labhart–Willi syndrome showing obesity.

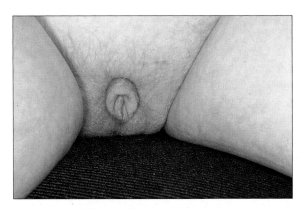

2.10 Prader–Labhart–Willi syndrome showing hypogonadism, age 14.5 years.

Features of the Prader–Labhart–Willi and Russell–Silver syndromes

Prader–Labhart–Willi

Short stature, usually from birth, certainly from mid-childhood, with small feet and hands
Early poor feeding and weight gain followed by overeating and obesity from early childhood
Almond shaped eyes and high forehead, squint
Hypotonia
Poor performance with behavior problems, especially related to food
Hypogonadism, osteoporosis, premature adrenarche
Diabetes mellitus (usually type 2, non-insulin dependent)
Partial deletion of the long arm of paternal chromosome 15, or evidence of maternal disomy

Russell–Silver

Small from birth with delayed bone maturation
Hemihypertrophy/atrophy
Clinodactyly
Small triangular lower face, the corners of the mouth may turn down
Mild blue sclerae
Thin or sparse head hair
Café au lait spots

2.11 Features of the Prader–Labhart–Willi and Russell–Silver syndromes.

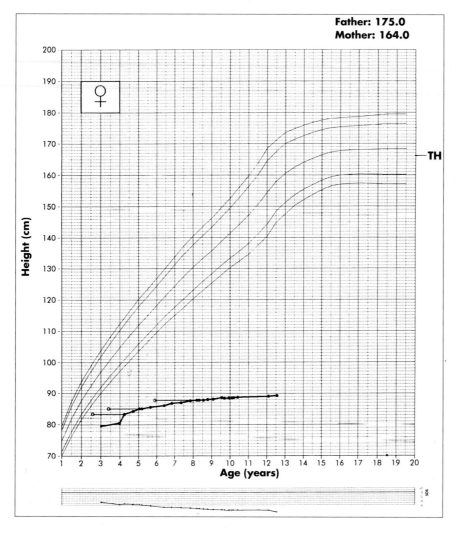

Father: 175.0
Mother: 164.0

2.12 Severe dwarfing as a result of a rare disorder, geleophysic nanism. Growth hormone was given between 6 and 7 years with no benefit. Death occurred at 13 years as a result of mitral valve involvement.

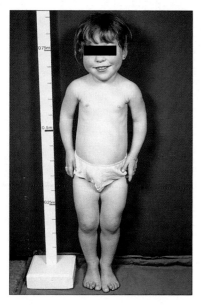

2.13 Severe primordial dwarfing (geleophysic nanism).

3. Intrauterine growth retardation (IUGR)

About 80% of children with intrauterine growth retardation or smallness-for-dates (a birth weight less than the 3rd centile for gestational age), attain a height and weight in the normal centiles within the first one or two years of postnatal life but fail to demonstrate catch up growth in height or weight. Asymmetrical IUGR with low birth weight but normal length is often caused by events late in pregnancy and usually has a good outcome. Symmetrical smallness (low weight and length) is less likely to recover and often hints at more severe, earlier or inherent problems, for instance:-

- genetic or metabolic disorders, e.g. chromosomal abnormalities and syndromes as described above including Russell–Silver (**2.11, 2.14**) and progeria (**2.15**).
- damage *in utero* by environmental agents (infections, drugs, alcohol) (**1.148**).
- growth potential permanently restricted by severe placental dysfunction (**2.16**).

4. Skeletal dysplasias

In general, body dimensions are abnormal in these disorders, mostly showing relatively short limbs. There is a spectrum of severity of relatively common short limbed dwarfing disorders from the severe achondroplasia to the milder hypochondroplasia, (**2.17–2.20**). The incidence of this group of disorders is around 1/15,000 live births. Achondroplasia is due to a single point mutation on chromosome 4p disrupting the fibroblast growth factor receptor causing poor division of bone-forming fibroblasts. It is likely that many of the other conditions in this spectrum share quantitatively and qualitatively similar defects.

In the various types of spondylo-epiphyseal dysplasia, spondylo-metaphyseal dysplasia (and the combined forms), the spine is affected along with specific areas of the long bones, producing variable shortening of the body segments and spinal deformity.

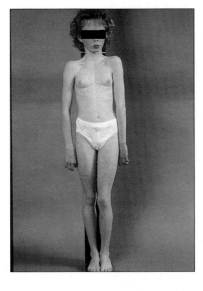

2.14 Russell–Silver syndrome. Previous history of low birth weight.

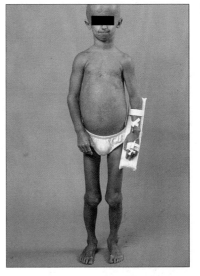

2.15 Progeria.

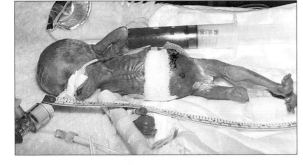

2.16 Severe smallness–for–dates (540 g) and prematurity (29 weeks), 60 ml syringe and tape measure for comparison. This combination of events has a poor eventual size prognosis.

There are also very many specific syndromes with bony dysplasia, some with dysmorphic features which overlap with those descibed above. The growth retardation seen in the Ullrich–Turner syndrome is considered by some to be due to an underlying skeletal dysplasia, providing further overlap. Some metabolic disorders affecting the bone, such as hypophosphataemic rickets may also be included in this group (**2.21**).

The diagnosis of these disorders is often difficult and may require expert radiographic review (see later). In general, there is no medical therapy even with a more specific diagnosis, but it can be important for prognosis and genetic counseling.

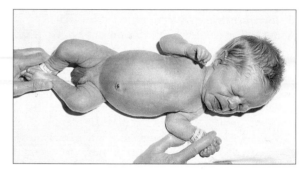

2.17 Achondroplasia at birth.

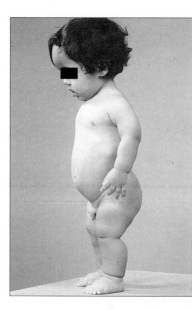

2.18 Achondroplasia age 2 years. Note trident hand.

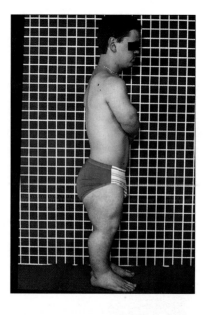

2.19 Moderately severe hypochondroplasia as young adult. Final height 125 cm (4 ft 1 in).

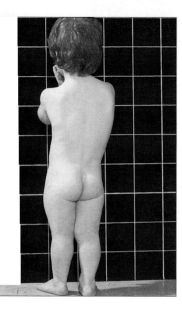

2.20 Mild hypochondroplasia presenting with disproportionate short stature (–3 SD).

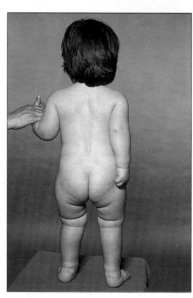

2.21 Hypophosphatemic rickets. Note extra skin creases on legs.

5. Storage disorders

These are rare and include mucopolysaccharidoses, mucolipidoses, and others that may have profound effects on the bony skeleton and other tissues. Of those which present primarily with short stature as opposed to their CNS or metabolic consequences, the most important are the Morquio syndrome (mucopolysaccharidosis Type 4) (**2.22**); mucolipidosis Type 3, which often presents first to rheumatologists because of the claw hands (**1.20**), and the juvenile form of the Hunter syndrome (mucopolysaccharidosis Type 2) (**2.23**), in which short stature and a large jaw may be the only presenting features before adult life when more severe complications ensue.

Glycogen storage disease Type 1a produces short stature with truncal obesity and thin limbs, a 'doll-like' face, hepatomegaly, and there may be macroscopic hyperlipidemia (**2.24, 2.25**). The other storage disorders present largely with neurological features.

Osteogenesis imperfecta (**2.26, 2.27**) and other disorders affecting collagen production such as the various Ehlers–Danlos syndromes may also be included in this category (**1.114, 1.134, 1.135**).

These disorders characteristically all have a major impact on the individual and there are also genetic implications. They are almost all characterized by a back that is relatively short when compared with the legs (**2.22, 2.23, 2.26–2.29**).

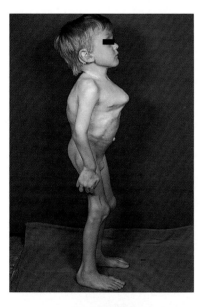

2.22 Morquio syndrome (mucopolysaccharidosis Type 4).

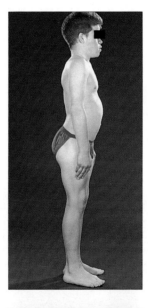

2.23 Juvenile Hunter syndrome (mucopolysaccharidosis Type 2). White cell enzyme assay showed zero activity of iduronosulfate sulfatase. Presented in mid-teens with short stature and noted to have prognathism and a short back (– 3.7 SD) compared to legs (– 2.5 SD) which led to the diagnosis.

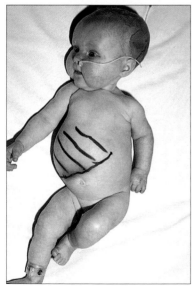

2.24 Glycogen storage disease Type 1.

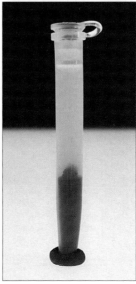

2.25 Macroscopic hyperlipidemia in same case as **2.24**.

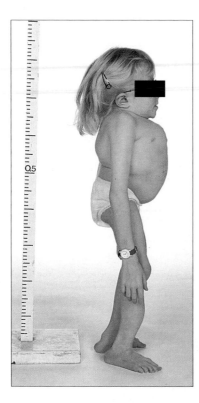
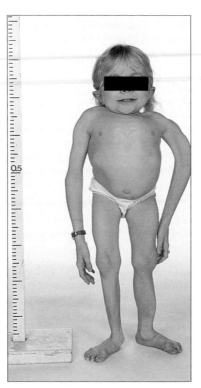

2.26, 2.27 Severe Type 3 osteogenesis imperfecta with shortening of back and limbs.

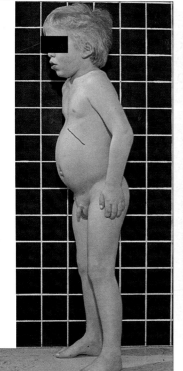
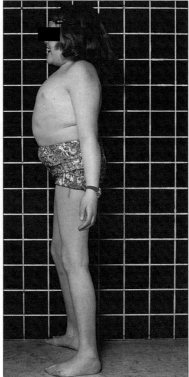

2.28, 2.29 Two cases of metabolic disorders (mucopolysaccharidoses 2 [**2.28**] and 4 [**2.29**]) emphasizing the relatively long legs when compared with the back.

SECONDARY GROWTH FAILURE

In this category there are five subgroups:

1. Disorders in specific systems
Disorders in specific systems including cardiac, lung, liver, intestinal, renal, hematological, CNS and generalized inflammatory disease. Often the diagnosis will have been made before the short stature is noted, however, even in the asymptomatic child, it is important to rule out hidden organic pathology. The dis-

orders that are most important to exclude are renal failure (**2.30**); chronic anemia; chronic infections (HIV, tuberculosis) and chronic inflammatory bowel diseases (e.g.Crohn's disease) (**1.88, 2.31**).

Gluten enteropathy (celiac disease) (**2.32–2.35**), in susceptible populations, may present very late in childhood (although it is more usual to present in infancy with anemia and failure to thrive) and have poor growth as its only feature. There may be abdominal distension and wasting of the buttocks but a high index of suspicion is required for the diagnosis.

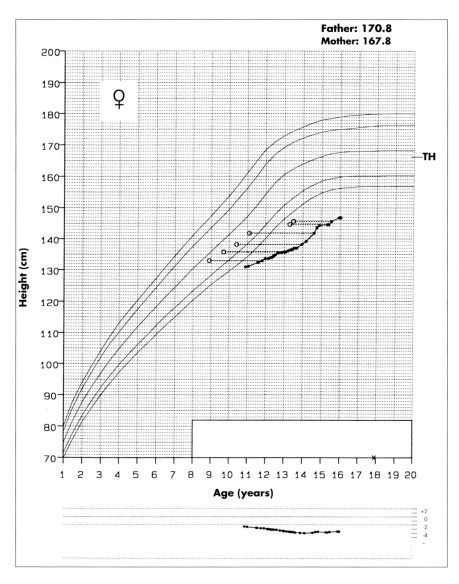

2.30 Age 10.9 years. Short stature (–2.5 SDS) and poor growth rate as presenting features of juvenile nephronophthisis causing renal failure. Treatment with estrogens was given to induce puberty at 14 years but the final height is much reduced (–4 SDS).

All of the above will tend to produce thinness (that may be even more pronounced than the short stature), or poor growth rate, documented as a weight centile below the height centile, no matter what the absolute height (or a reduced weight-for-height on a weight-for-height chart).

Diencephalic syndrome is a rare association of anterior hypothalamic tumors and extreme cachexia, usually presenting in early childhood (**2.36–2.39**). There is often hyperkinesia and there may be later associated endocrine abnormalities (see below).

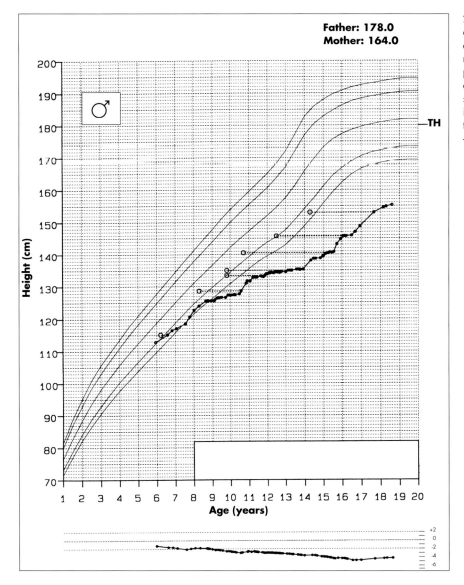

2.31 Crohn's disease diagnosed at six years of age (–1 SDS). No growth response to hemicolectomy, parenteral nutrition or elemental diet. Pubertal spurt, 16.5–18.5 years, induced by depot testosterone but final height –4 SDS.

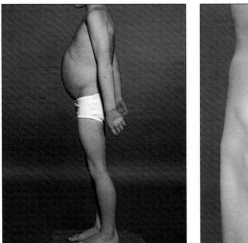
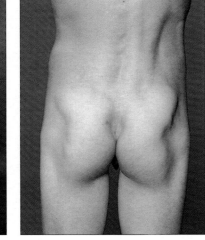

2.32, 2.33 Late onset celiac disease with abdominal distension and wasting of the buttocks.

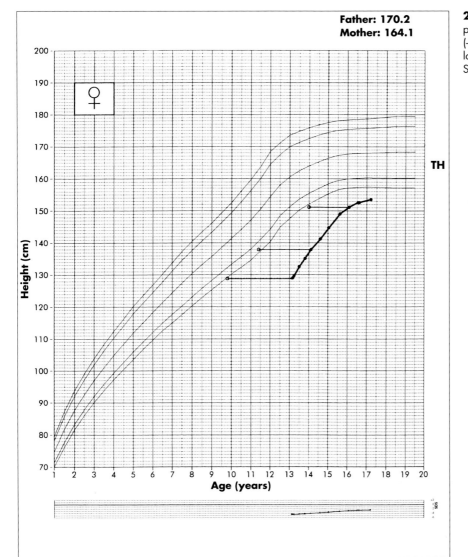

Father: 170.2
Mother: 164.1

TH

2.34 Gluten enteropathy presenting as short stature (–4.8 SDS) at 13.2y, with later catch-up growth to –2.4 SDS on gluten free diet.

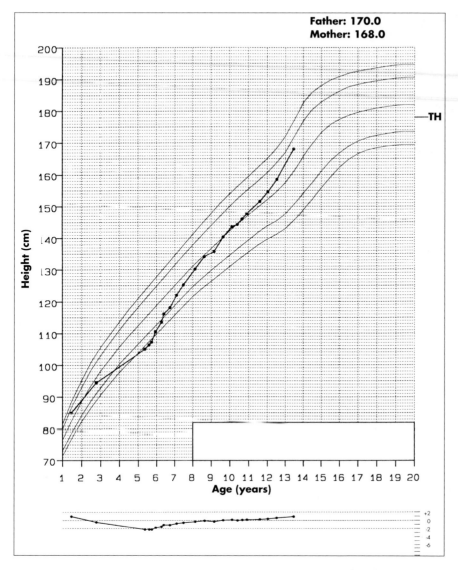

Father: 170.0
Mother: 168.0

2.35 Gluten enteropathy presenting at 5.5 years (–2.2 SDS) with later complete catch-up on gluten free diet to within the target range.

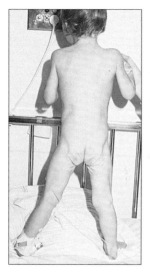

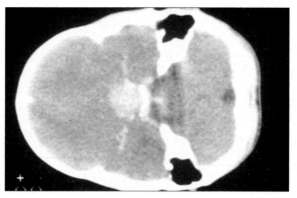

2.36, 2.37 Diencephalic syndrome, CT scan of the associated optic glioma.

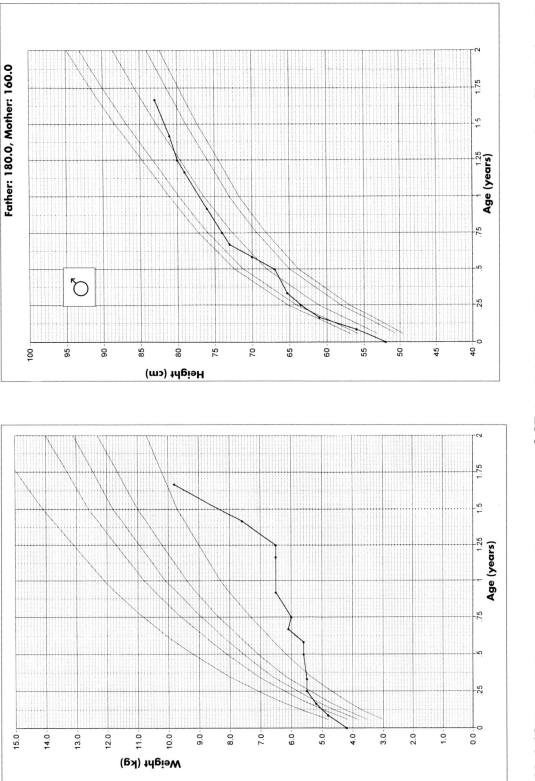

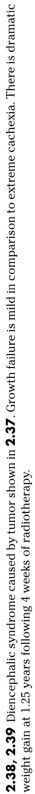

2.38, 2.39 Diencephalic syndrome caused by tumor shown in **2.37**. Growth failure is mild in comparison to extreme cachexia. There is dramatic weight gain at 1.25 years following 4 weeks of radiotherapy.

Endocrine disorders

The main endocrine disorders causing short stature in children are hypothyroidism, GH deficiency, pseudo-hypoparathyroidism and the Cushing syndrome. Rarely, poor regulation of blood sugar in a diabetic child can lead to short stature (Mauriac syndrome). (**2.40, 2.41**). Patients with hypogonadism (see chapter 5) can be short in the pubertal age range. Relative obesity is often a feature of all of these conditions.

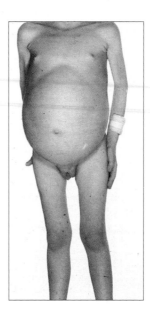

2.40 Mauriac syndrome showing limb wasting and distended abdomen secondary to hepatomegaly. Height SDS was more than -3 SD and puberty was delayed.

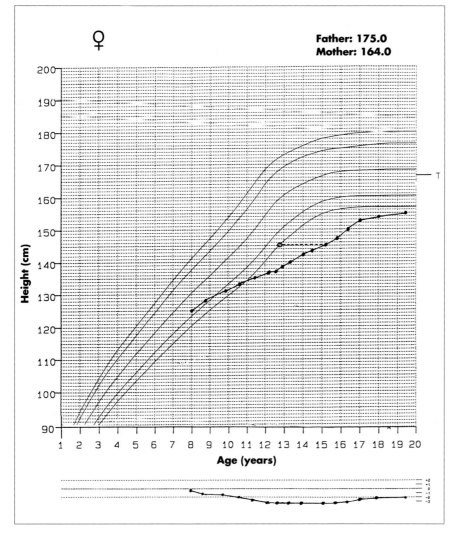

2.41 Growth chart of Mauriac syndrome showing loss of height potential and delayed puberty in poorly controlled diabetic.

Hypothyroidism

Untreated congenital hypothyroidism (**2.42**) (see Chapter 7) which is less commonly seen since the advent of neonatal screening, produced a final height similar to severe growth hormone deficiency.

In the much more common acquired hypothyroidism (**2.43**) there is growth retardation with obesity and delayed skeletal maturation and dentition. Usually puberty is delayed (Chapter 5), but can be precocious with lactorrhea (Chapter 4). The cause in iodine sufficient areas is usually an autoimmune thyroiditis, but it may occur in response to therapeutic irradiation. Isolated central hypothyroidism is rare (see Chapter 7).

Growth hormone deficiency

Growth hormone deficiency (GHD) may indeed be complete, for instance in familial gene deletion cases or after surgical removal of the pituitary gland with craniopharyngioma. It is more often a relative lack that may be defined in terms of response to various provocation tests or from the frequency and amplitude of overnight secretory episodes. The more minor degrees of deficiency merge with the lower end of the normal range and idiopathic short stature.

Unequivocal GHD from an early age historically produced an adult height of between 130–140 cm (around 4 feet 5 inches or approximately –5 SD below the population mean) (**2.44**) and was not uncommon, (estimates vary between 1/4,000 to 1/20,000 of the population depending on the definition of severity). It may still present late with markedly short stature (**2.45**), but more commonly presents with relatively mild short stature and a slow rate of growth. There is relative obesity (**2.46**). The increasing number of survivors of childhood malignancy who have received

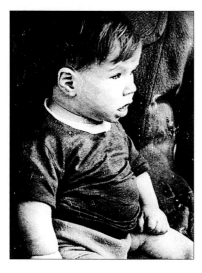

2.42 Cretinism. Untreated congenital hypothyroidism.

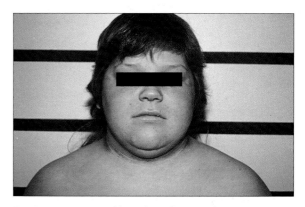

2.43 Gross acquired hypothyroidism.

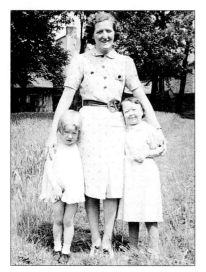

2.44 Classical growth hormone deficiency. Normal 2 year old in comparison to mother and 50 year old affected aunt.

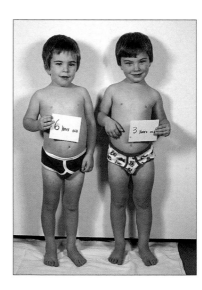

2.45 Growth hormone deficiency in a 6 year old with sibling aged 3 years.

cranial irradiation and have subsequently developed GHD means that this will be the commonest cause of GHD by the end of the century (**2.47**).

Growth hormone generates a mediator, insulin growth factor-1 (IGF-1) or somatomedin-C, at local cartilage level to promote bone growth. Circulating levels of IGF-1 are dependent on hepatic synthesis and may not affect the growth process directly. The various genetic mutations in the GH receptor that prevent generation of IGF-1 produce the rare Laron syndrome where there is clinical GHD in the presence of normal or high GH levels and undetectable IGF-1 (**2.48, 2.49**).

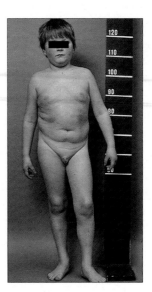

2.46 Obesity in isolated growth hormone deficiency.

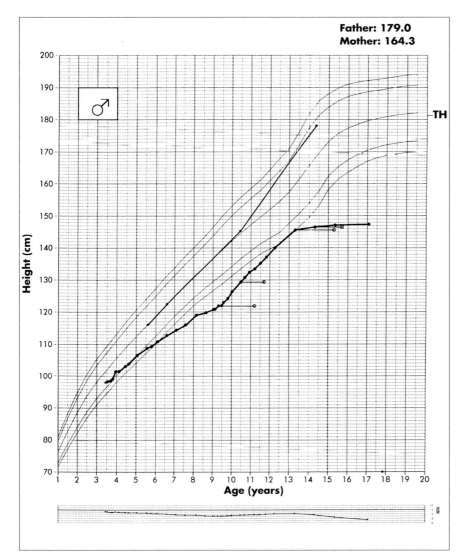

Father: 179.0
Mother: 164.3

2.47 Severe growth retardation (final height –5 SDS) secondary to chemotherapy and irradiation for a bone marrow transplant in ALL. There was growth hormone deficiency and diabetes mellitus (both treated from 9.25 years) as well as hypo-thyroidism (from 12 years). Gonadotropin secretion was not affected. The height of the donor identical twin is shown (light line) to illustrate the development and magnitude of the height loss in the patient.

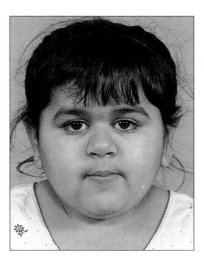

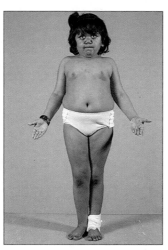

2.48, 2.49 Laron syndrome, facial view and whole body. Note obesity and mid-face hypoplasia. The possibility now exists for treatment of the short stature with recombinant IGF–1.

Pseudohypoparathyroidism

This is a rare heterogeneous disorder of post receptor activation where variable hypocalcemia is associated with moderate short stature, obesity, 'moon-face' and shortening on the metacarpals, (most often the IVth (**1.28, 1.29, 2.50**) with cone shaped epiphyses). The hypocalcemia is resistant to treatment with PTH and may result in learning difficulties, cataracts and ectopic calcification. Primary hyperparathyroidism and central hypogonadism may coexist. [The differentiation between pseudo- (with hypocalcemia), and pseudo-pseudohypoparathyroidisim (without hypocalcemia), has been abandoned as the hypocalcemia is variable and both types have been described in the same family].

The Cushing syndrome

Other than being caused by the administration of topical, oral, inhaled or injectable steroids the Cushing syndrome is rare in childhood. The causes are summarized in (**2.51**) . Very little excess cortisol or other steroids are required to inhibit growth, hence growth failure is almost universal (except in rare cases of adrenal tumor where testosterone production predominates causing a 'pubertal' growth pattern). The most striking feature of hyperadrenocorticism is a rapid increase in body fat (**2.52–2.54**), particularly the abdomen, the face ('moon face') (**2.55, 2.56**) and the cervical fat pad ('buffalo hump') (**2.57**). A thinning of the skin causes striae which are especially prominent in the iatrogenic syndrome (**2.58**) and capillary

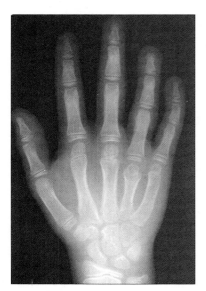

2.50 Short fourth metacarpal in child with hypocalcemia.

Causes of the Cushing syndrome in childhood and adolescence, in order of frequency

Iatrogenic
Pituitary adenoma (most common in late childhood)
Adrenal adenoma (most common in early childhood)
Adrenal carcinoma
Bilateral nodular hyperplasia
Ectopic ACTH production

2.51 Causes of the Cushing syndrome in childhood and adolescence, in order of frequency.

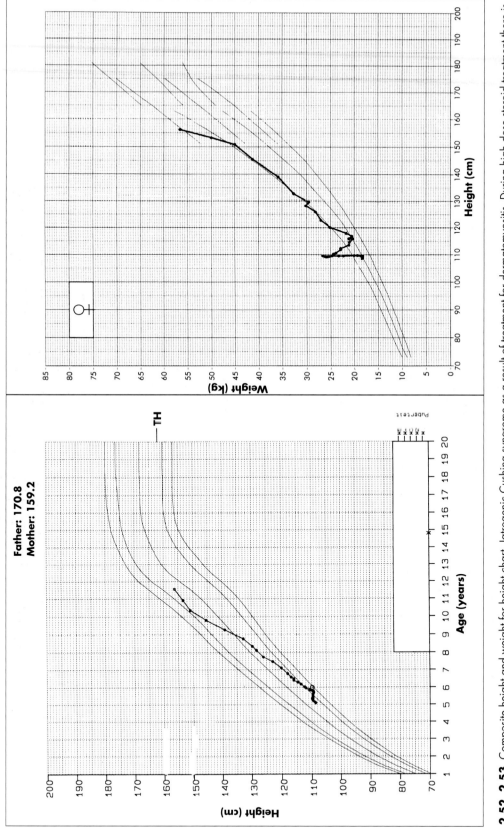

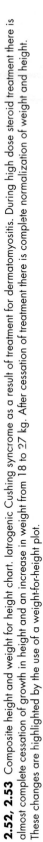

2.52, 2.53 Composite height and weight for height chart. Iatrogenic Cushing syncrome as a result of treatment for dermatomyositis. During high dose steroid treatment there is almost complete cessation of growth in height and an increase in weight from 18 to 27 kg. After cessation of treatment there is complete normalization of weight and height. These changes are highlighted by the use of a weight-for-height plot.

friability leads to ecchymoses. There is weakness and a decreased muscle mass, but this appears less striking in children than in adults. Hypertension is usually, but not always, present. Demineralization of bones occurs, but is not often clinically detectable. In non-iatrogenic forms of the syndrome the secretion not only of glucocorticoids, but also of androgens, is increased, and signs of hyperandrogenization (excessive hair, acne, cliteromegaly) may be present.

In adulthood the differentiation of nutritional obesity from the Cushing syndrome may be difficult, but in childhood, although some of the features may be similar (**2.59**), the relative tall stature associated with overeating means that there is seldom diagnostic confusion.

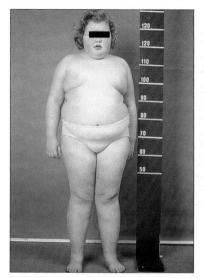

2.54 Cushing disease due to pituitary adenoma. Gross obesity.

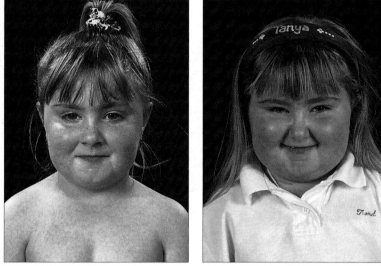

2.55, 2.56 Progression from mild to severe Cushingoid facies in child with unresectable adrenal adenoma.

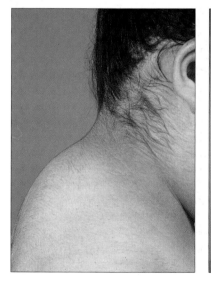

2.57 Cushing syndrome with buffalo hump and hirsutism.

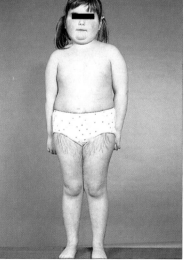

2.58 Iatrogenic Cushing syndrome secondary to treatment for dermatomyositis.

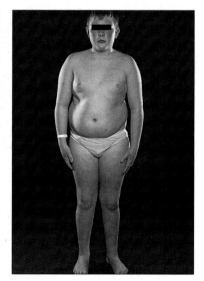

2.59 Pseudo-Cushing syndrome secondary to nutritional obesity. Note high cheek color. There was hypertension and skin fragility. Height was however on 95th centile. Urinary free cortisol was normal and there was later a supra-normal rate of growth.

3. Metabolic disorders

Many inborn errors of metabolism are associated with short stature but present primarily with neurological or signs in other systems.

The Bartter syndrome of hypokalemic alkalosis may present with failure to thrive, vomiting and constipation in early infancy.

4. Iatrogenic short stature

This may be either as a result of treatment of childhood malignancy or caused by glucocorticoid treatment. The dose of steroids that may produce growth failure is far less than that needed to produce the other features of the Cushing syndrome and any child on steroids, either topical, inhaled or oral should have his or her growth regularly monitored (**2.60**).

5. Psychosocial short stature

Psychosocial short stature, also called emotional or psychosocial dwarfism, is caused by an extremely poor emotional environment. Although there is usually relative thinness, this is not always the case and there can be considerable diagnostic confusion between deprivation dwarfism and GHD. The GH response to stimulation testing can be severely, but reversibly, blunted and there is diminished spontaneous overnight GH secretion. There is a lack of response to GH therapy and a rapid catch-up seen on a change of care-giver (**2.61, 2.62**). There is commonly a preservation of infantile body proportions (**1.136**).

More minor degrees of short stature are a consequence of more minor deprivation, which may contribute to the well known social class gradient in height.

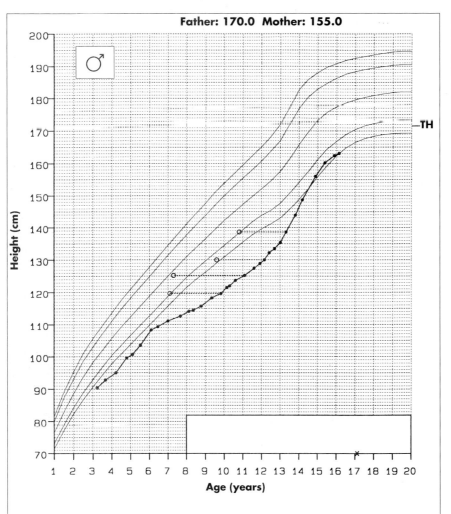

2.60 Growth failure secondary to treatment with inhaled beclomethasone dipropionate, 200 mg twice a day from 6 to 12 years of age. There is also constitutional short stature which led to the clinical presentation of this case. Final height is within the target range.

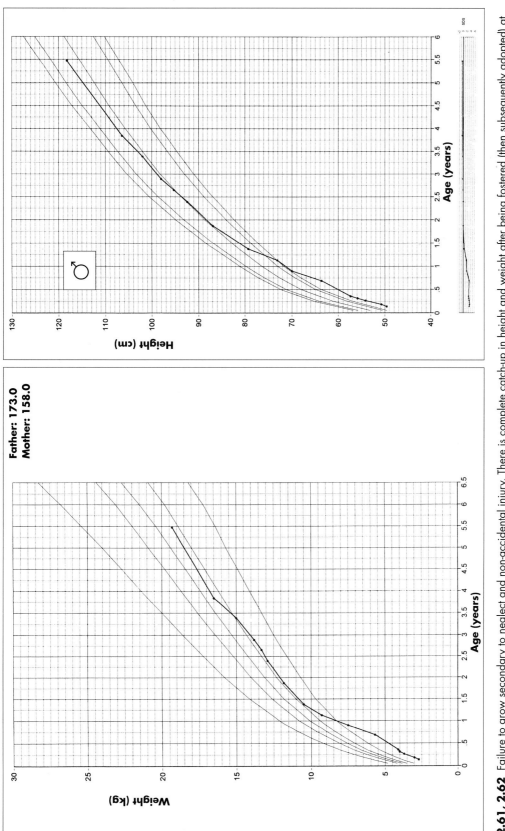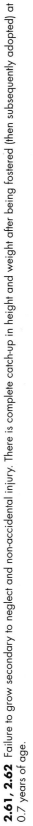

Father: **173.0**
Mother: **158.0**

2.61, 2.62 Failure to grow secondary to neglect and non-accidental injury. There is complete catch-up in height and weight after being fostered (then subsequently adopted) at 0.7 years of age.

DIAGNOSTIC WORK-UP OF SHORT STATURE

MEDICAL HISTORY AND PHYSICAL EXAMINATION

The following are the most relevant points to include when taking the history of a child presenting with short stature (also see Chapter 1).
- The pattern of growth in height and weight. Include birth weight and length (in relation to duration of pregnancy).
- The presentation at birth (breech delivery is associated with growth hormone deficiency and many syndromic disorders).
- Parental heights: calculate the target height and compare its centile position with the patient's height centile. (Beware the dominantly inherited relatively mild disorders of growth that may be undiagnosed in one parent, such as hypochondroplasia.)
- Family history: ask about the onset of puberty of the mother (age at menarche) and father (late onset? – the father may remember that he continued to grow in late teenage life or shaved later than his friends).
- Milestones of puberty in the patient: (onset of breast development, menarche; onset of penile enlargement, pubic hair).
- Nutritional assessment.
- Previous diseases and operations.
- Drug administration including inhaled and topical preparations, over-the-counter medication and herbal remedies.
- Neurological symptoms (especially headache and disturbance of vision).
- Gastrointestinal, pulmonary, cardiac, urogenital symptoms.
- Psychosocial situation.

A full physical examination has to be performed, with special emphasis on the following:
- Accurate measurements of height, weight, sitting height, head circumference. Other special measurements may be required.
- Calculate the ratio between sitting height and leg length and compare this to reference values.
- Nutritional state, fat distribution – skinfold thickness if possible.
- Pubertal stage.
- Dysmorphic stigmata in the hands, feet, head and neck etc.
- Heart, lungs and abdomen to exclude other organic diagnoses.
- A neurological examination (including fundoscopy and visual fields (**1.107, 1.108**). The relaxation of the Achilles tendon reflex is slow in hypothyroidism.

Hypotonia and developmental delay are a feature of some dysmorphic syndromes.
- Skin signs.
- Palpation of the thyroid gland (see Chapter 7).

INTERPRETATION OF THE CLUES

If height is below the 3rd centile and no physical abnormalities are found, there are several possibilities:
- Height is concordant with the target height centile = familial short stature unless a parent has a demonstrable pathology.
- Height is discordant with parental height = CDGA, idiopathic short stature or mistaken paternity.
- Isolated growth hormone deficiency and late presenting coeliac disease may be very silent in their manifestations.

Clues which point to one of the primary growth disorders include:
- Specific dysmorphic features and/or mental retardation = one of the syndromic causes of short stature.
- Low birth weight and length for gestational age = intrauterine growth retardation with failure to catch up.
- Body disproportion. a) Legs < back = skeletal dysplasias. b) back < legs = disorders of bone metabolism, spondyloepiphyseal dysplasia and storage disorders (but also to a more minor degree can be seen in delayed puberty for whatever cause).
- Hypogonadism = the Ullrich–Turner syndrome, Prader–Labhart–Willi syndrome.

Pointers to chronic disease are:
- Specific signs in any system.
- Low growth rate / short stature accompanied by thinness.
- Anemia.

Pointers to an endocrinopathy include:
- A history of breech position and prolonged jaundice. The finding of a low height velocity, frontal bossing, increased abdominal fat, delayed puberty and a high-pitched voice = growth hormone deficiency (± signs of an additional pituitary deficiency).
- Low height velocity, obesity, sparse hair, discordant pubertal development, delayed bone age, irregular or heavy periods, constipation, goitre, pre-tibial myxedema, slow relaxation of the Achilles tendon reflex = hypothyroidism.
- Low height velocity, sudden rapid weight gain with a centripetal distribution, hirsutism, hypertension, weakness, glycosuria, striae, bruising and moon face = the Cushing syndrome.

RADIOLOGICAL AND LABORATORY INVESTIGATIONS

If the clinical assessment and analysis of the growth curve indicate a pathological growth pattern, further investigations are warranted. In such cases a radiograph of the left hand and wrist for bone age should always be performed. Other investigations should be aimed at confirming or ruling out the most likely diagnoses (See Appendix B for normal values and diagnostic test procedures).

Disproportion present

- In cases with body disproportion or obvious skeletal abnormalities a limited skeletal survey should be performed. (**2.63–2.72**).
- If a storage disorder is likely then several urine specimens should be collected for analysis of mucopolysaccharides and consideration should be given to an assay of white cell enzyme levels – a simpler screening test may be to ask for examination of a blood film looking for vacuolation of lymphocytes.
- Serum calcium, phosphate and alkaline phosphatase are measured to evaluate bone diseases. Assays of collagen metabolites or genetic studies may be available in specialist centers.

Proportionate short stature

If no body disproportion is present, a short screening programme can be carried out (**2.73**), consisting of:

- Full blood count with MCV. Anemia may be present especially in inflammatory bowel disease, celiac disease and renal failure although it can be present in almost any prolonged illness. Microcytosis is an indication of nutritional deficiency and blood loss and macrocytosis may indicate malabsorption.
- Acid base status, urea and electrolytes, creatinine, liver function, calcium, phosphate and alkaline phosphatase. This will exclude occult renal failure and hepatic disease, the Bartter syndrome and metabolic bone disease.
- Urine analysis (simple biochemistry and microscopy).
- Stool analysis (giardiasis can produce profound growth retardation and may be picked up only if the stool is inspected microscopically for cysts). Test for reducing substances to exclude lactose intolerance. The presence of red blood cells and fat globules may point towards celiac disease and the need for a jejunal biopsy.
- TSH ± FT4 (free T4 levels are preferable to total T4 levels as they are not prone to interference with drugs, renal or hepatic disease (see Chapters 7 and 8)).
- IGF-1 and IGFBP-3 (see below).
- Antigliadin antibody screen.
- Chromosome analysis.

Proportionate short stature with relative overweight

If GH-deficiency is suspected further testing of the GH - IGF-1/ IGFBP-3 axis should be performed. Normal levels of IGF-1 or IGFBP-3 largely exclude GH deficiency. Low levels may be due to several causes, including nutritional inadequacy and do not prove GH deficiency, hence a GH provocation test should be performed at an experienced center (see Appendix B).

Radiographs to be taken as part of a limited skeletal survey

Lateral skull
Chest
Lateral lumbar spine
Hips and pelvis including lower lumbar spine
Left hand and wrist (also for bone age)
One long bone (tibia or fibula the best)
Forearm bones if any limitation of movement or external abnormality

2.63 Radiographs to be taken as part of a limited skeletal survey.

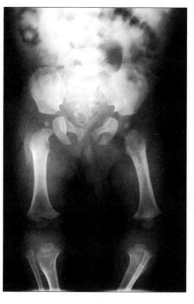

2.64
Achondroplasia. Short tubular bones, metaphyseal flare, square 'beaked' pelvis.

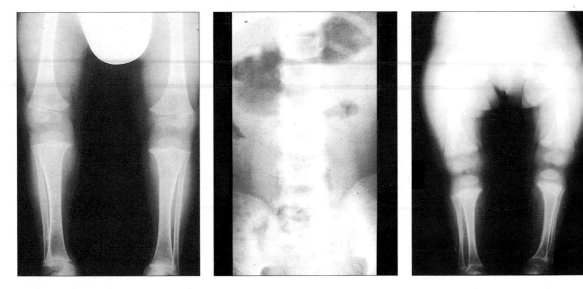

2.65, 2.66 Hypochondroplasia. Less marked shortening of bones than in achondroplasia, fibula relatively long, lack of widening of the lumbar interpeduncular distance.

2.67 Hypophosphatemic rickets.

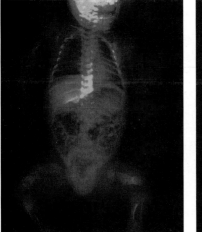

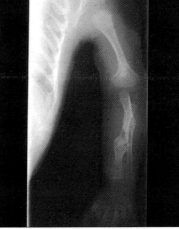

2.68, 2.69 Severe Type 3, autosomal recessive, and the common (80% of all cases) Type 1 dominantly inherited osteogenesis imperfecta.

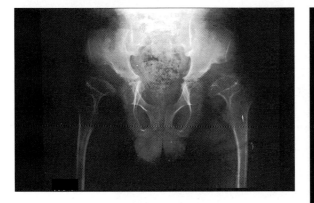

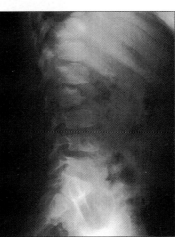

2.70, 2.71 Dysostosis multiplex with abnormal beaked vertebra in mucolipidosis 3.

Plain skull x-rays may show abnormalities suggestive of raised intracranial pressure or craniopharyngioma (**2.74**), but may also be normal and are thus unreliable as a primary investigation. Magnetic resonance imaging or computerized tomography is thus advisable in all cases of proven deficiency to exclude craniopharyngioma (**2.75, 2.76**), or other tumors (**2.77**) and document anatomical abnormalities such as empty sella, ectopic pituitary tissue or stalk disruption (**2.78–2.80**).

In the Laron syndrome there is a failure to generate IGF-1 in response to normal or high levels of GH.

The commonest forms of hypothyroidism may be detected by raised TSH in the preliminary screen. If found this should prompt assay of anti-thyroid antibody levels. Isolated central hypothyroidism is rare but will be detected by the low-normal TSH level at the same time as a low free T4. Further details of thyroid function testing are given in Chapter 7 and Appendix A.

If the Cushing syndrome is suspected an estimation of 24h urinary free cortisol (UFC) should be obtained followed by a serum cortisol rhythm (early morning, 0700–0900 and 2200–midnight) and a simultaneous measurement of ACTH. Suppression of ACTH implies an adrenal cause. Raised cortisol levels, UFC and loss of diurnal variation should prompt referral to a specialist center for further evaluation with dexamethasone testing (see Appendix A), and localization of the source by MRI scanning of the pituitary or CT scanning of the abdomen and chest (**2.81**). Sampling for ACTH from the inferior petrosal sinus can help lateralize pituitary adenomas in 60–70% of cases where scanning is equivocal, in experienced units.

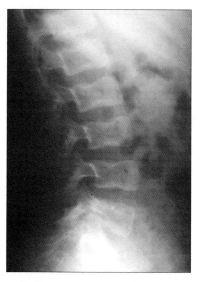

2.72 Platy-spondyly in spondylo-metaphyseal dysplasia.

Suggested brief screening program for the investigation of proportionate short stature

Full blood count and film
Renal and liver function tests, calcium / phosphate,
  alkaline phosphatase and acid-base status
Urinalysis
Stool analysis for fat globules, Giardia cysts,
  red blood cells, etc
Thyroid stimulating hormone ± FT4
IGF-1 and IGFBP-3
Antigliadin antibodies
Chromosome analysis

2.73 Suggested brief screening program for the investigation of proportionate short stature.

2.74 Plain skull radiograph of craniopharyngioma. There is erosion of the posterior clinoid process and suprasellar calcification. The plain radiograph may be normal, however, and should not be relied upon in the investigation of short stature or hypopituitarism.

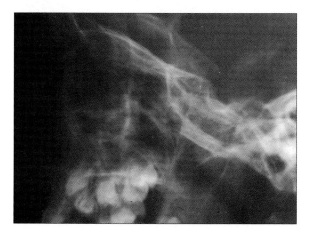

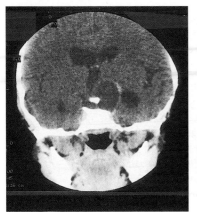

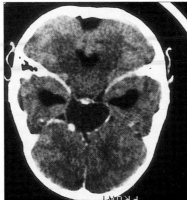

2.75, 2.76 Vertical and horizontal CT scans of a cystic craniopharyngioma with calcification.

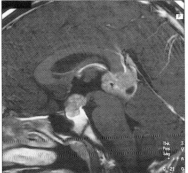

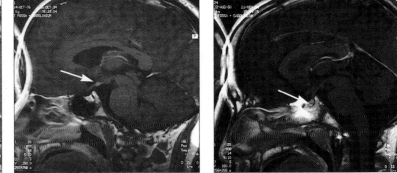

2.77 MRI scan of bifocal germinoma (pineal and pituitary) presenting with panhypopituitarism.

2.78, 2.79 MRI scan showing ectopic pituitary tissue as a bright spot anterior to the mammillary bodies (left arrow). Normal MRI scan for comparison shows pituitary stalk, posterior pituitary bright spot (right arrow).

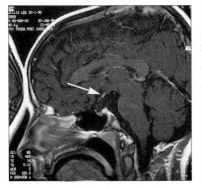

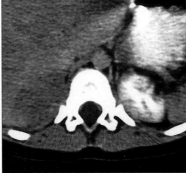

2.80 MRI scan showing evidence of damage to the pituitary stalk in a child with multiple anterior pituitary hormone deficiencies. ADH gives a bright signal and can be seen 'held-up' in mid-stalk at the site of presumed damage.

2.81 CT scan of right sided adrenal adenoma producing the Cushing syndrome. The hypo-dense tumor has displaced the right kidney downwards, the left kidney is outlined with contrast medium.(Same case as **2.34**.)

THERAPY OF SHORT STATURE

Idiopathic and primary short stature

Treatment of these conditions remains both experimental and controversial and should remain in the realm of the specialist centers. Growth hormone treatment should still be offered as only part of a formal clinical trial except possibly in the Ullrich–Turner syndrome where there is currently the only convincing evidence for benefit on final height in any of the primary disorders (**2.82**). The GH dose is 1.0 u/kg/week – approximately 0.3 mg/kg/week – given as a daily subcutaneous injection. Anabolic steroids such as oxandrolone (dose 0.06 mg/kg/day) may have an added benefit.

In idiopathic short stature there may be early acceleration of growth rate, but a shortened duration of growth, and there is currently no evidence to suggest that final height is increased.

In the skeletal dysplasias, surgical leg lengthening techniques in specialist units (**2.83–2.85**) offer the possibility of height gain in the order of 10–25 cm, (4–10 inches). The use of medical growth promoting therapies is being explored, but are likely to be of lesser importance than surgery.

In the storage disorders, there may be a role for bone marrow transplantation to reduce the metabolic and skeletal consequences of the underlying defect. There is some evidence that the skeletal, if few of the other, symptoms of these conditions can at least be stabilized by this procedure.

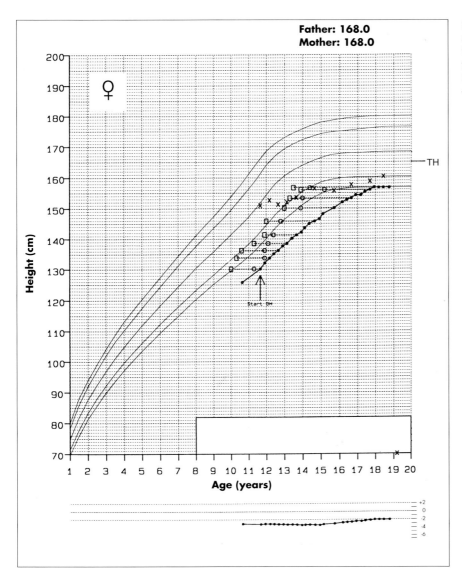

2.82 The Ullrich–Turner syndrome. Growth hormone therapy initiated at 11.8 years. There is an improvement in height from –3 to –2 SDS.

Secondary growth failure

If the growth failure is due to a systemic illness, successful treatment of the specific systemic disorder may produce catch-up growth. This is particularly true of disorders that are active in late childhood and early teenage life where even a relatively brief period of amelioration of a disease process may allow for a more normal pubertal growth and an increased height prognosis.

Growth hormone deficiency is treated with daily subcutaneous administration of synthetic growth hormone at a dose of 0.5–0.7 u/kg/week, approximately equivalent to 0.15–0.25 mg/kg/week (**2.86, 2.87**). Laron syndrome may be treated with recombinant IGF-1 in specialized centers.

Treatment of the Cushing syndrome is always highly specialized. If due to an adrenal adenoma it is treated by unilateral adrenalectomy. Adrenal carcinomas are highly aggressive and combined medical and surgical treatment is required for any hope of success. Pituitary adenomas causing Cushing disease may be treated with trans-sphenoidal adenomectomy followed by temporary adrenal replacement therapy till adrenal function recovers. If resection of the pituitary adenoma is not possible, and in cases of the syndrome caused by bilateral nodular adrenal hyperplasia, then bilateral adrenalectomy may be required [but at the risk of causing the Nelson syndrome (**1.129**)], followed by lifelong replacement therapy with gluco- and mineralocorticoids.

Hypothyroidism is easily treated with L-thyroxine tablets at a dose tailored to suppress the TSH level, usually between 50 and 150 µg/day. The catch-up growth that might be expected from the degree of skeletal immaturity that is present at diagnosis may not occur, especially if the growth failure is long-standing or occurs during puberty (**2.88**).

The Bartter syndrome may be treated with a combination of salt supplements, potassium sparing diuretics and indomethacin.

Psychosocial deprivation dwarfism may show impressive catch-up if it is possible to change the circumstances of care (**2.61, 2.62**). Recovery of height and weight gain whilst separated from the usual carers can be used as retrospective evidence of the nature of the problem.

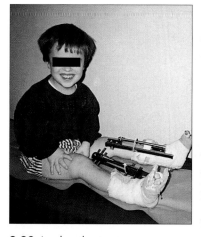

2.83 Leg lengthening in achondroplasia with bilateral tibial fixators.

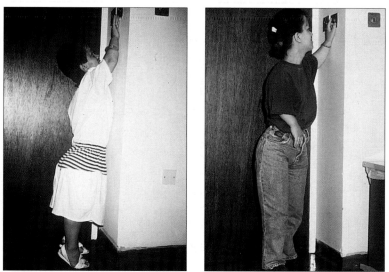

2.84, 2.85 Results of leg lengthening in achondroplasia after 2 year program of tibial and femoral lengthening. Before surgery unable to reach lightswitch, after surgery a gain of 28 cm.

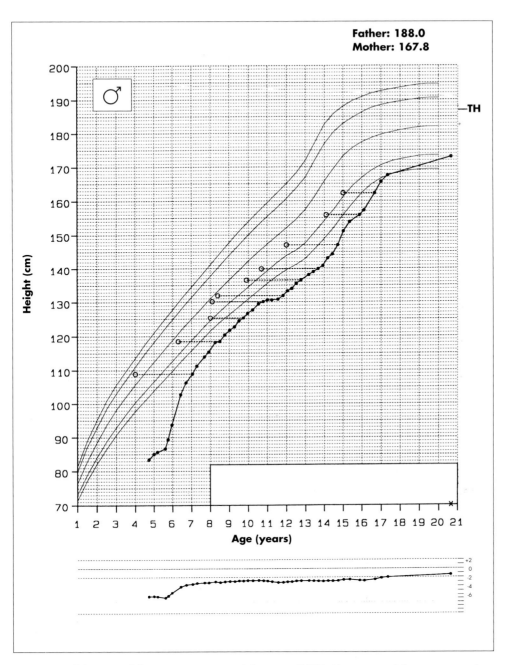

Father: 188.0
Mother: 167.8

2.86 Growth hormone deficiency presenting at 4.8 years; –7 SDS. Human growth hormone started at 5.8 years with height gain to –3 SDS. Human growth hormone discontinued at 11 years with cessation of growth for 6 months before re-institution of recombinant GH therapy, given three times a week. Changed to daily therapy at 14 years with further acceleration of height velocity. Depot testosterone used to induce puberty at 16 years of age. Final height –1.8 SDS.

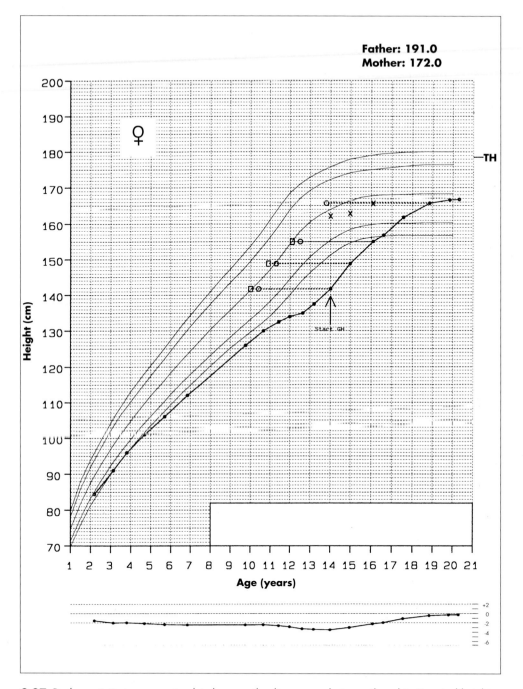

Father: 191.0
Mother: 172.0

2.87 Panhypopituitarism presenting late because the discrepancy between the subject's actual height (–2 SDS, at the bottom of the normal range through late childhood) had not been interpreted in the context of the tall parents (target height +1.8 SDS). Thyroxine and hydrocortisone started at 13.2 years, recombinant GH at 14 years and ethinylestradiol at 16 years. Final height –0.2 SDS; below target height but within normal range.

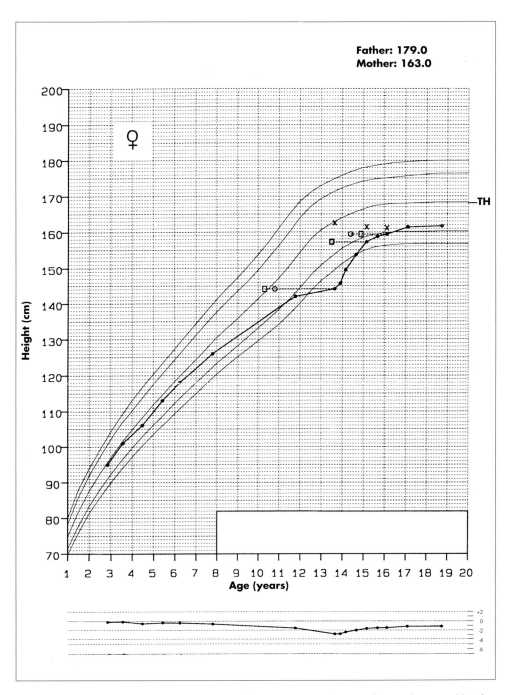

Father: 179.0
Mother: 163.0

2.88 Hypothyroidism presenting at 13.8 years of age (–3 SDS) with incomplete catch-up. Final height –1 SDS, below target range; previous height prior to hypothyroid state –0.2 SDS.

3.

The Large Child

AETIOLOGY

The classification of causes of tall stature, with or without obesity, is more straightforward than that of short stature. Idiopathic or genetic tall stature is by far the commonest cause. There are a relatively small number of primary syndromes of large size and secondary causes of increased final height are rare. Some secondary conditions produce largeness for a period of the child's growth span, then a normal or even reduced final height. There are also primary disorders of blood supply or intrinsic to the growth plate that can produce areas of localized overgrowth.

IDIOPATHIC TALL STATURE

Idiopathic tall stature is defined by the absence of abnormalities in the history and physical examination. It can be subdivided in the same way as for short stature, described in Chapter 2.

1. **Familial tall stature, characterized by:**
- Tall stature during the growth period and an increased final height.
- A normal height velocity (varying around the 75th centile)*.
- A height within the range defined by parental size, although doubtful paternity may sometimes cause confusion.
- Bone age consistent with (±2SD) chronological age.
- A normal age of onset of puberty.

- Often relatively long legs compared to sitting height.
*[As the height centile lines diverge with increasing age a tall child on the 97th height centile will show a velocity that varies around the 75th velocity centile.]
2. **Constitutional early puberty, characterized by:**
- Normal to tall stature during childhood.
- Final stature within the range defined by parental size.
- A moderately advanced bone age (not more than +2SD above chronological age).
- An increased height velocity (>75%) in the later childhood years.
- Early onset and cessation of puberty, often following the same pattern as one or both of the parents.
3. **A combination of both conditions is often seen.**
4. **Tall stature plus nutritional obesity.**
In adult endocrine practise the differentiation between secondary endocrine and primary nutritional causes of obesity may be difficult. In childhood the extra calorie intake is available for growth and so may produce relatively tall stature characterized by:
- Tall stature (at upper end of predicted target range), with weight ≥ height centile (**3.1**).
- Relatively early puberty.
- Striae and high cheek color mimicking mild Cushing syndrome (**3.2**) but with the contrasting rapid growth compared with the almost universal growth failure of steroid excess.
- Frequently a similar habitus in one or both parents and siblings.

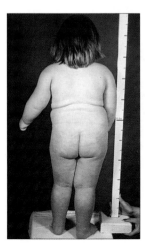

3.1 Nutritional obesity, height >97%; 15 kg (33 lb) overweight for height at age 3 years.

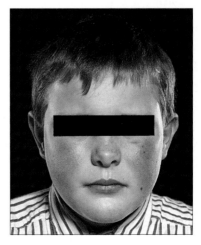

3.2 High cheek color mimicking Cushing syndrome in nutritional obesity.

PRIMARY CAUSES OF LARGE SIZE

There are four broad categories:

1. Proportionate large size plus intellectual deficit

There are several syndromes associated with tall stature and mental retardation:
- Sotos syndrome (**3.3–3.7**).

- Weaver syndrome (**3.8**).
- Marshall–Smith syndrome.
- Beckwith–Wiedemann syndrome (**3.9–3.11**) which includes macrosomia (often more marked on one side of the body), with other dysmorphic features and hypoglycemia. There may be associated intellectual deficit as a result of the hypoglycemia.

The main distinguishing features of these conditions are given in (**3.12**).

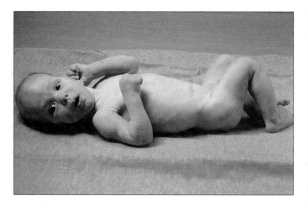

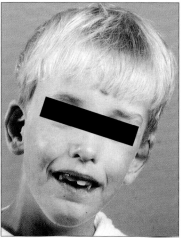

3.3–3.5 Sotos syndrome as baby, child and young adult (185 cm, 6ft 1in).

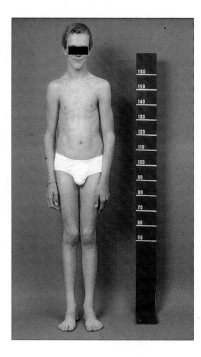

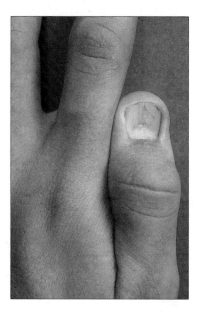

3.6 Deep-set concave nails in Sotos syndrome.

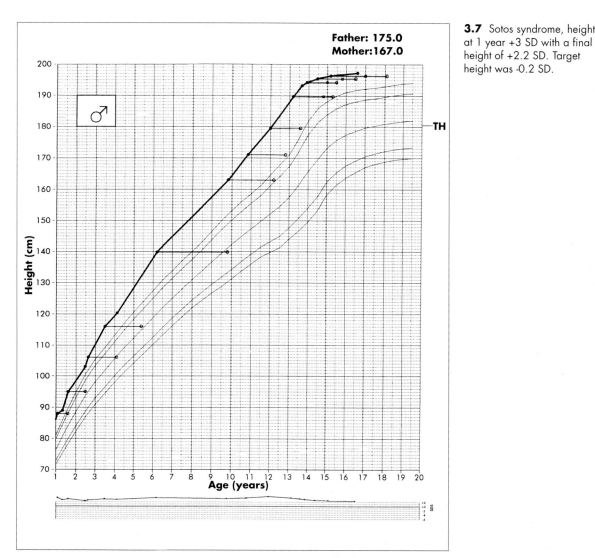

Father: 175.0
Mother: 167.0

3.7 Sotos syndrome, height at 1 year +3 SD with a final height of +2.2 SD. Target height was -0.2 SD.

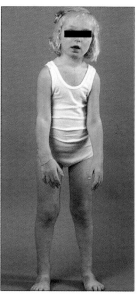

3.8 Weaver syndrome, height >97%.

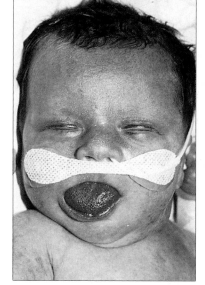

3.9 Facial features of Beckwith–Wiedemann syndrome.

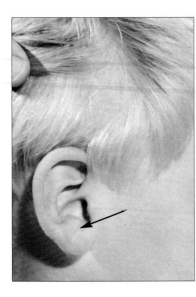

3.10 Beckwith–Wiedemann syndrome. Demonstration of ear crease.

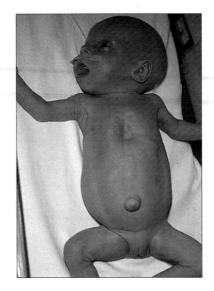

3.11 Beckwith–Wiedemann syndrome, showing umbilical hernia and abdominal distension from organomegaly.

Features of the major syndromes associated with large size

	Beckwith–Wiedemann	Sotos	Weaver	Marshall–Smith
Head and face				
	Big at birth	Big at birth	Variable	Ht > Wt
	Large muscle mass till teens	Growth rate slows after 4y	Flat occiput	Bone age *very* advanced
	Prominent occiput	Prominent forehead	Macrocephaly	Prominent forehead
	Facial hemangiomas	Macrocephaly	Large ears	Long head
	Ear lobe crease	Hypertelorism, squint	Micrognathia	Big nose
	Small mid-face	Prognathism	Thin head hair	Shallow orbits
	Macroglossia	Early teeth, narrow palate	Hypertrichosis	Hypertrichosis
IQ and CNS				
	Hypoglycemia, which may cause secondary IQ reduction	Abnormal GTT Mild/moderate primary	Primary IQ reduction IQ reduction	Primary IQ reduction Myopathy
Other				
	Organomegaly	Deep set nails	Hoarse voice Nail hypoplasia	Blue sclerae
	Hemi-hypertrophy	Hernias	Stiff joints Camptodactyly	Reduced immunity
	Cardiac defects	Cardiac defects	Cardiac defects	Cardiac defects
Tumors				
	Wilms tumor Hepato-, neuro-, gonado-blastomas	Wilms tumor Vaginal, hepatic, parotid and neuro-ectodermal carcinomas	Neuroblastoma	?

3.12 Features of the major syndromes associated with large size (see also **3.3–3.11**).

2. Disproportionate tall stature with normal intellect

- The Marfan syndrome is a relatively common dominantly inherited disorder of one of the copies of a fibrillin gene on chromosome 17q. It is characterized externally by disproportionate tall stature (**3.13**) with relatively long legs (**3.14**), arachnodactyly (**3.15**), joint laxity (**1.17, 1.18**), hernias, scoliosis and chest deformities (**1.81, 1.82**), myopia, dislocation or poor fixation of the lens (**1.113**) and a high arched palate (**1.64**). Internally, there may be weakness of the collagenous structures, especially on the left side of the heart producing mitral and aortic valve incompetence, aortic dilatation and dissection. Spontaneous pneumothorax may occur.

- Beals contractual arachnodactyly (**3.16**) is a rare dominantly inherited disorder of another copy of a fibrillin gene on chromosome 15q and has some similarities with the Marfan syndrome. There are contractures at the knees, elbows and hands and micrognathia. The ears may be 'crumpled' and there may be kyphoscoliosis.
- Multiple endocrine adenomatosis or neoplasia (MEA or MEN) type 2b is a familial condition where the occurrence of medullary carcinoma of the thyroid and pheocromocytoma is associated with mild tall stature and a marfanoid habitus (**3.17**) along with neuromas of the mucous membranes (**1.66**).
- Hypogonadism can cause a modestly increased final height with long legs (the so-called

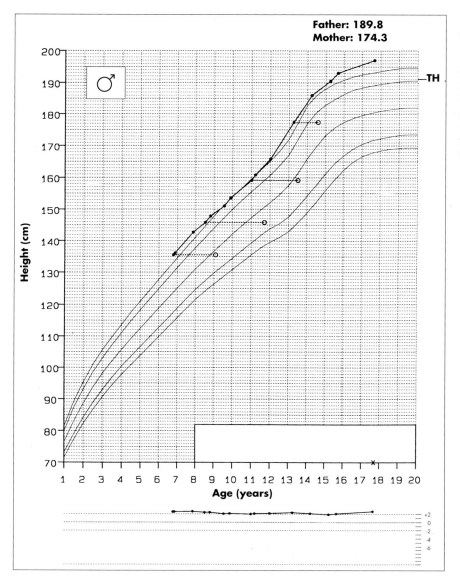

Father: 189.8
Mother: 174.3

3.13 The Marfan syndrome occurring as a new mutation. Note the normal parental heights. Moderate tall stature (final height +2.5 SD but not outside target range), with a slightly early pubertal spurt. Final sitting height and leg length SD were +1.8 and +3.0 respectively.

'eunuchoid body habitus'), on the basis of late closure of the epiphyses and prolonged childhood growth of the legs coupled with failure of the sex-hormone mediated growth of the spine (**3.18**). The causes and work-up of hypogonadism are discussed in Chapter 5.

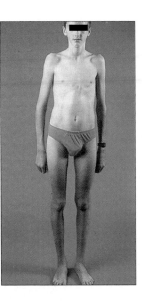

3.14 The Marfan syndrome.

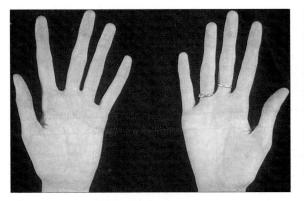

3.15 Arachnodactyly in the Marfan syndrome.

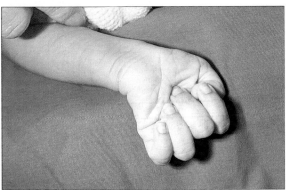

3.16 Beals contractural arachnodactyly.

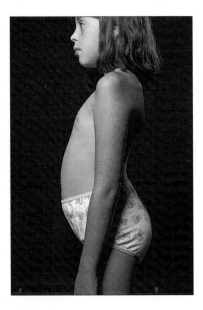

3.17 Multiple endocrine adenomatosis type 2b, marfanoid habitus.

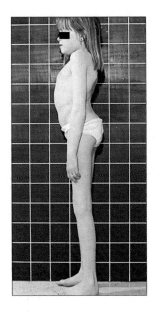

3.18 Extreme eunuchoid body habitus (legs>>back).

3. Disproportionate tall stature plus intellectual deficit

Many abnormalities involving duplication of the X or Y chromosomes can occur, but only two are commonly associated with disproportionate tall stature, the Klinefelter (XXY, XXYY, XXXY and mosaic forms) and the XYY syndromes. In both the legs are relatively long compared to the back (**3.19**).

- The Klinefelter syndrome is most commonly associated with the XXY karyotype, but variants with XXYY and mosaic forms can occur. (An XXXY form is more likely to be associated with slow growth.) There tends to be minor intellectual deficit, often exacerbated by behavioral problems and hypergonadotrophic hypogonadism. In later life there is a high incidence of diabetes mellitus.

- XYY males have a mild intellectual deficit and specific motor co-ordination problems. In the past it was said that there was an increase in antisocial behavior, but this is not now thought to be commonly the case. Cryptorchidism occurs but is not as universal as in the Klinefelter syndrome. Both conditions are relatively common, occurring more than twice as frequently as the Ullrich–Turner syndrome in birth karyotype surveys, however, the relatively mild learning difficulties and the social acceptability of tall stature mean that they often present in late childhood or early adult life.

- Homocystinuria is an aminoaciduria that is associated with marfanoid tall stature (**3.20**), but will more frequently present because of the ocular complications such as ectopia lentis (**1.113**) and severe myopia. Intellect is usually subnormal and complications associated with thromboembolism occur.

4. Local overgrowth syndromes

Hemihypertrophy is most commonly associated with overall short stature (as in the Russell–Silver syndrome, see Chapter 2), and with the Beckwith–Wiedemann syndrome (see earlier). However, isolated growth of one or more limbs (and organs such as the penis) can occur secondary to abnormal lymphatic and venous supply and is called the Klippel–Trenaunay–Weber syndrome (**3.21**, **1.123**).

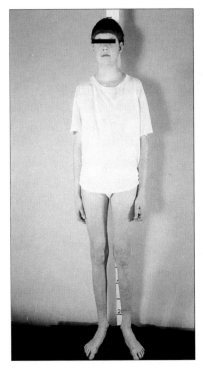

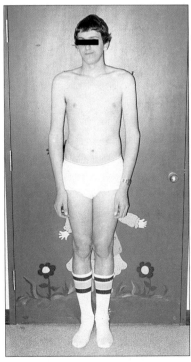

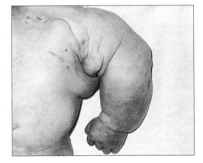

3.21 Klippel–Trenaunay–Weber syndrome secondary to lymphangioma.

3.19 XXY, final height (with treatment) 208 cm (7 ft).

3.20 Homocystinuria, 190.5 cm (6 ft 3 in) at 13.5 years.

SECONDARY CAUSES OF LARGE SIZE

Infancy

Intra-uterine hyperinsulinemia secondary to maternal diabetes (**3.22, 3.23**) or pancreatic endocrine dysregulation (nesidioblastosis) (**3.24**) (see Chapter 8) causes early macrosomia as insulin is a potent fetal growth factor. This increase in size is usually transient and followed by 'catch-down' growth once the abnormal insulin secreting environment is removed.

Childhood

Other causes of large size are rare and include pituitary gigantism, thyrotoxicosis and sexual precocity. Hypothalamic tumors may produce pathological obesity and secondary tall stature.

- Pituitary gigantism (**3.25–3.27**) is extremely rare. It is produced by growth hormone excess caused by a GH-producing adenoma in the pituitary. Proportionate, worsening tall stature with an elevated height velocity is seen and if no treatment is given can produce heights in excess of 200 cm. The same disease process produces acromegaly in adulthood after the fusion of the epiphyses and a number of patients with a late childhood onset share many features of both conditions. There may be prognathism and signs and symptoms due to optic chiasm compression. There may be increased sweating and a yellowish discoloration of the palms (**1.45**).

- Thyrotoxicosis (see also Chapter 7) (**3.28, 3.29**), if mild and hence unrecognized and untreated, produces an acceleration of growth rate and relative tall stature in mid-childhood, although there is advanced osseous maturation and the eventual height is liable to be in the genetic range.

- Precocious puberty is discussed in detail in Chapter 4 and leads to tall stature in childhood, but not a tall final height. Untreated, the increasingly advanced bone age leading to early epiphyseal fusion means that final height is usually reduced.

- Hypothalamic tumors producing overeating with obesity are a rare secondary cause of tall stature (**3.30**).

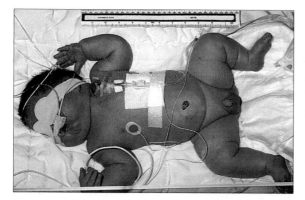

3.22 Infant of a diabetic mother. Macrosomia, plethora and jaundice requiring exchange transfusion.

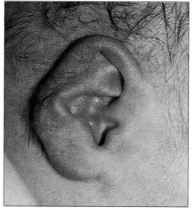

3.23 Hairy ears in the infant of a diabetic mother.

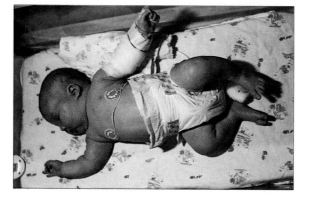

3.24 Neonatal hyperinsulinism secondary to pancreatic endocrine dysregulation syndrome (nesidioblastosis).

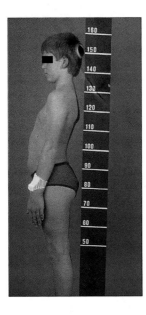

3.25 Pituitary gigantism, 160 cm (5 ft 3 in), aged 9 years, prepubertal. Chart shown below.

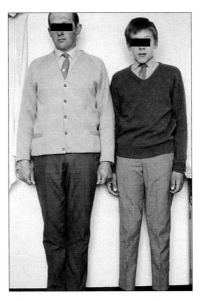

3.26 Pituitary gigantism, age 9 years, in comparison to father.

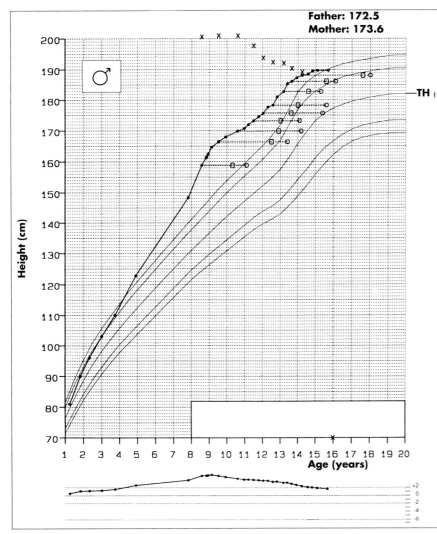

Father: 172.5
Mother: 173.6

3.27 Pituitary gigantism presenting as tall stature (+5 SD) at 9 years of age with evidence of previous accelerating height velocity. Adenoma resected at 9.2 years with fall in SD to a final height of +1.8. Testosterone given from 11.5 years.

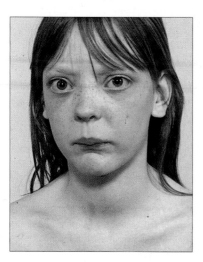

3.28
Thyrotoxicosis.

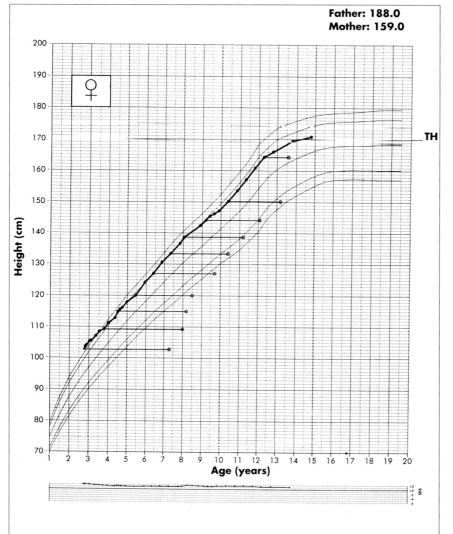

3.29 Thyrotoxicosis
presenting at 2.8 years with
a bone age of 7.4 years
and height of +2SD.
Subsequent growth on
antithyroid therapy for 4
years, followed by eventual
remission, was normal (final
height +1SD).

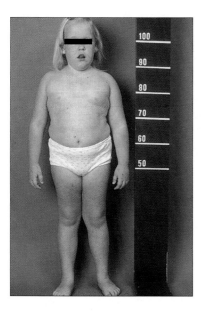

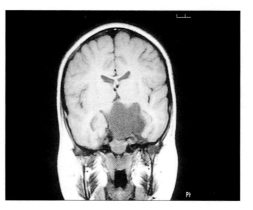

3.30, 3.31 Obesity with MRI scan of arachnoid cyst in same case.

DIAGNOSTIC WORK-UP OF TALL STATURE

MEDICAL HISTORY AND PHYSICAL EXAMINATION

The following are the most relevant points to explore when taking a history of a child presenting with large size:–
- Birth size, mother's health and gestational history, mode of delivery.
- Parental size and timing of puberty.
- Any family history of early heart disease or eye problems.
- Any symptoms suggestive of early sexual development.
- Any symptoms of sweating, tremor, frequent stool habit, anxiety or heat intolerance.
- Dietary intake.
- Neurological symptoms including headache and visual disturbance. Is the sense of smell normal? (Anosmia is associated with hypogonadism in the Kallmann syndrome – see Chapter 5.)
- Developmental or educational level. Any specific motor or behavioral defects?

On examination look especially for:–
- The pattern of growth of height, sitting height, weight and head circumference. The presence or absence of disproportion is an important feature. Head circumference is large in Sotos syndrome and as the height SDS stabilizes after 2 years of age patients become less noticeably tall.
- Horizontal skin striae on the back, often seen in rapidly growing tall individuals for whatever cause (**3.32**).
- Dysmorphic features as outlined in (**3.12**).
- Neuromas, enlarged thyroid or hypertension (paroxysmal initially), in MEN 2b.
- Any evidence of hypogonadism or cryptorchidism.
- Plethora and hairy ears which are seen in infants of diabetic mothers.
- Discoloration of the palms.
- Visual field deficit, optic disc appearance and the position of the lens.
- Goitre, tremor, exophthalmos or other signs of thyrotoxicosis.

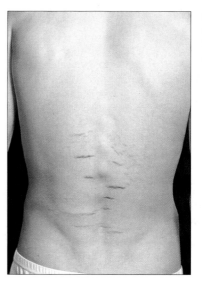

3.32 Horizontal striae in idiopathic tall stature.

INTERPRETATION OF THE CLUES

The absence of any physical abnormalities or disproportion with no evidence of sexual precocity indicates:
- If Wt ≤ Ht centile = familial tall stature.
- If Wt > Ht centile, (or abnormal (>97%) weight-for-height plot) = nutritional.

Large size with specific dysmorphic features and intellectual defect:
- = one of the overgrowth syndromes (**3.12**).

Disproportion with normal intellect:
- With arachnodactyly = the Marfan or Beals syndrome. There may be no family history if a new mutation has occurred.
- With only moderate tallness, neuromas on lips, tongue or eyelids (**1.66, 3.17, 3.33**), and a positive family history (although new mutations occur frequently) = MEN type 2b.
- With moderate tall stature, hypogonadism and anosmia = the Kallmann syndrome.
- With moderate tall stature and hypogonadism = isolated or iatrogenic (i.e. following irradiation), hypogonadism.

Disproportion with intellectual defect:
- If hypogonadism or cryptorchidism = X chromosome duplication.
- If ocular and neurological problems predominate = homocystinuria.

Enlargement of one side of body or one limb:
- If associated with dysmorphic features as shown in **3.12** = Beckwith–Wiedemann syndrome.
- If associated with haemangioma = Klippel–Trenaunay–Weber syndrome.

Large size with no disproportion:
- If present at birth = neonatal hyperinsulinism.
- If accelerating height velocity, neurological signs of optic chiasm compression, sweatiness, prognathism or skin signs = pituitary gigantism.
- If goitre, exophthalmos, tremor, tachycardia = thyrotoxicosis.
- If early sexual development (less than 8 years in a girl, less than 9 years in a boy) = precocious puberty.

RADIOLOGICAL AND LABORATORY INVESTIGATIONS

These are less commonly required than in the investigation of short stature.

A hand and wrist radiograph for bone age will serve the dual purpose of providing an estimation of physiological maturity and allow quantification of arachnodactyly.

The bone age is mildly advanced in familial tall stature/early puberty and more so in precocious puberty and thyrotoxicosis. The bone age is very advanced in the Marshall–Smith syndrome and less so in the other dysmorphic overgrowth syndromes. In the Weaver syndrome only the maturation of the carpal bones is in advance of the small bones of the hand.

A metacarpal index compares the average length to width ratios of the metacarpal bones in an attempt to define arachnodactyly as a value of > 8.5. In practice it adds little to an external clinical assessment. In the presence of genital abnormalities the karyotype should be checked.

If there is any possibility of MEN 2b either because of a positive family history or the presence of mucosal neuromas in a child with a marfanoid habitus it is essential rapidly to check the calcitonin level and urinary VMA level, and refer the child to a specialist for a pentagastrin stimulation test as the implications for missing an early diagnosis of medullary cell carcinoma of the thyroid are so severe.

Neonatal hyperinsulinism in infants born to non-diabetic mothers can be confirmed by the demonstration of inappropriately high insulin levels at the time of hypoglycaemia.

If suspicion exists then thyroid function tests (to demonstrate a suppressed TSH level) or urine estimation of homocystine levels are indicated. The assessment of sexual precocity is described in Chapter 4 and hypogonadism in Chapter 5.

If pituitary gigantism is a possibility then an elevated IGF-1 level may be a useful screening test followed either by a physiological GH profile (**3.34**) or the demonstration of a failure of suppression of GH levels to a glucose load (see Appendix A).

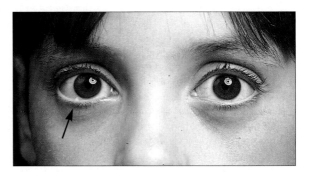

3.33 Neuroma on right lower eyelid in MEN IIb.

THERAPY

The treatment of children to limit their final height is a highly specialized area that should be confined to experienced centers.

In idiopathic tall stature a likely final height of more than 185 cm (6 ft 1 in) in a girl or 200 cm (6 ft 6½ in) in a boy may be arbitrarily defined as 'excessive', although much depends on the psychological adjustment of the child and support from parents and peers. It is a mistake to treat children because of abnormal perceptions of tallness or past adverse experiences of one or both parents.

Artificial induction of an accelerated puberty will serve to limit final height to a degree. This is usually performed by administering high daily doses of oral ethinyloestradiol (100–200 micrograms) to girls and depot injections of testosterone (up to 500 mg every 2 weeks) to boys. Associated with this therapy are the psychological problems of a sudden entry into sexual maturity and the physical ones of tender breasts and genitalia and a sudden onset of acne etc. Priapism in boys on depot testosterone and thromboembolism in girls on estrogen treatment have been described. The future risks of long term side effects, especially in girls of families with a strong history of breast cancer, are unknown but of concern.

Trials of recombinant long acting somatostatin analogue treatment are in progress and offer a more physiological approach to therapy but the long-term results of this treatment are still unknown.

There is probably no justification for treating the majority of those affected by the primary over-growth syndromes as final height is seldom cosmetically a problem.

It is often stated that sex hormone treatment of the Marfan syndrome should be approached with caution as there may be theoretical risks of increasing the likelihood of early cardiovascular disease, although published data to support this contention are lacking.

If a diagnosis of MEN 2b is made there should be urgent referral for prophylactic thyroidectomy, followed by thyroxin, vitamin D and calcium replacement therapy and lifelong surveillance for the development of pheocromocytoma.

Boys with X duplication will need testosterone replacement therapy initiated in order to undergo secondary sexual development and minimize disproportion. Conventionally this is performed using depot testosterone injections (50–100–250 mg sequentially – see Chapter 5 for details), although patches, oral preparations and gonadotrophin therapies may be used in some centers. All these treatments may worsen behavior problems.

The results of treating the hemangiomas associated with local overgrowth are very poor. Surgical resection of long bone segments have been attempted to reduce height in various tall stature syndromes, but with limited success and a high morbidity. The treatments of sexual precocity, hypogonadism and thyrotoxicosis are discussed in Chapters 4, 5 and 7 respectively.

Basal tumors causing obesity should be referred to a specialist paediatric neurosurgeon for assessment and treatment. Likewise the trans-sphenoidal resection of a pituitary adenoma requires great expertise.

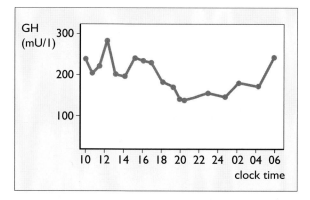

3.34 Growth hormone profile in pituitary gigantism.

4.

Early Sexual Development

HORMONAL CHANGES IN PUBERTY

The earliest biochemical event of puberty is the appearance of intermittent serum peaks of luteinizing hormone and follicle stimulating hormone at night, caused by a pulsatile secretion of gonadotropin releasing hormone (GnRH) from the hypothalamus. The pituitary GnRH receptors are responsive only to pulsatile GnRH; continuous administration blocks the secretion of gonadotropins. The intermittent production of LH and FSH stimulates the gonads leading to sex hormone secretion and the development of the germinal epithelium. Initially the sex hormones are elevated only for part of the day.

In the male the enlargement of the testes from a prepubertal 3 ml volume to 4 ml heralds the onset of puberty as the Sertoli cell volume increases. It is possible to have functioning Leydig cells and testosterone secretion in damaged testes (for instance after irradiation) without a volume increase. Testicular testosterone (via target cell conversion to dihydrotestosterone; see Chapter 6) produces pubic hair and penile growth and is slightly augmented by androgen secretion from the adrenal gland. Acne, mood swings, the breaking of the voice, attainment of an adult body odor and sweat pattern are all androgen mediated events.

In the female the first external sign of puberty is an enlargement of the breast bud as estrogen is produced from the ovary. Some of the androgen-mediated effects seen in a girl, including pubic and axillary hair growth, are secondary to increased androgen secretion from a maturational change in the adrenal gland – adrenarche. Adrenarche occurs in both sexes but is usually subsumed in the male by testicular androgen production. In the female, along with some ovarian-derived androgens, adrenarche forms an important component of normal pubertal development.

Cyclical LH and FSH production leads to ovarian enlargement, follicle production and ultimately to maturation of the uterus and endometrium, followed by menarche. These changes can be monitored by ultrasonography (**4.1–4.4**).

Peripheral aromatase conversion of testosterone to estrogen, especially by fatty tissue, is possible and is responsible for estrogen-mediated breast enlargement, gynecomastia, in some males.

Neonates are exposed to the maternal hormone environment and may manifest changes secondary to natural or iatrogenic hormone exposure. Withdrawal bleeding in females (**4.5**) and neonatal breast enlargement (**1.91**) in both sexes are physiological results of this process. Additionally there is a physiological activation of the hypothalamic-pituitary-gonadal axis in the first months of life, especially in boys, which then subsides till puberty (**4.6**).

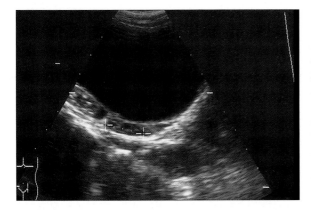

4.1 Ultrasonic demonstration of the internal age-related changes in uterus and ovaries (**4.1–4.4**). After the neonatal period the ovaries are small (long axis 18 mm +–+ in this section), and contain only one tiny follicle.

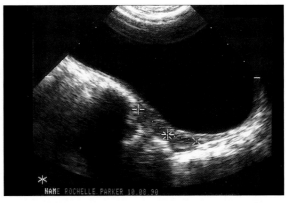

4.2 The pre-pubertal uterus is small (16 mm long +–+) and tubular and not steeply angled in relation to the cervix (13 mm long x–x).

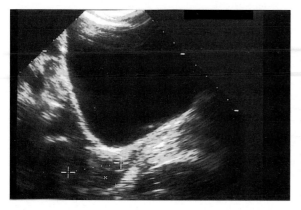

4.3 At puberty the ovaries enlarge (here 35 mm long +–+) and contain larger, peripheral follicles (one here measured 9 mm x–x). Through the menstrual cycle one such follicle will become dominant, enlarge till ovulation then regress to form a corpus luteum.

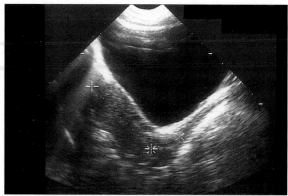

4.4 The late pubertal uterus is clearly pear shaped (61 mm long +–+) and contains a mid-line endometrial echo. It is steeply angled in relation to the cervix (22 mm long x–x) and the vagina can be clearly seen extending upwards to the right.

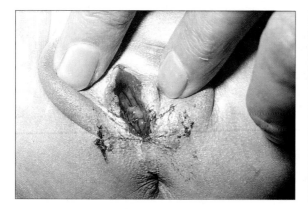

4.5 Physiological withdrawal bleeding in a neonate.

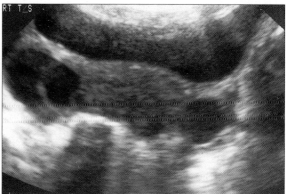

4.6 Transverse section of neonatal pelvis. The uterus is the solid mid-line structure behind the bladder. Both ovaries contain large follicles secondary to physiological neonatal activation of the hypothalamo-pituitary-ovarian axis

CLASSIFICATION OF EARLY PUBERTY

Early or precocious puberty (also called sexual precocity) is defined by the onset of puberty before 8 years (girls) or 9 years (boys). It can be subdivided into 'true' (or 'central') precocious puberty and 'pseudo' sexual precocity. True precocious puberty is all of the events of normal puberty occurring early, whereas in pseudo-precocious puberty only some aspects of sexual development occur, depending on whether androgens or estrogens are produced. Excess or early estrogen production in the female or testosterone in the male leads to iso-sexual development. Alternatively excess or early estrogen produc-

tion in the male or testosterone in the female leads to heterosexual development

There are also two forms of partial development, which are usually considered as variations of normal: premature adrenarche/pubarche (early pubic hair) and premature thelarche (breast development). (Note that as the first sign of true precocious puberty in a girl is breast development, the differentiation between early puberty and premature thelarche cannot be made only on the basis of a single physical examination. One must consider both growth pattern and bone age which are normal in premature thelarche and accelerated in precocious puberty, as well as the progression of sexual development.)

TRUE SEXUAL PRECOCITY (CENTRAL PRECOCIOUS PUBERTY)

This is characterized by:
- Concordant development of all structures usually involved in puberty: in a girl breast then pubic hair growth (**4.7**) and uterine and ovarian maturation followed by menarche; in a boy testicular enlargement, penile and pubic hair growth (**4.8**).
- The simultaneous development of secondary effects such as mood swings, acne (**4.9, 1.100**), body odor.
- A pubertal height spurt (**4.10**).
- Advanced bone age which continues to progress rapidly and leads to premature epiphyseal closure and hence reduced final height.

True sexual precocity can be idiopathic (by far the most frequent form in girls) or caused by abnormalities in the central nervous system (most commonly in boys). These can be congenital anomalies, hypothalamic hamartomas (**4.11**), elevated intracranial pressure, or tumors (**4.12**), and can follow cranial irradiation especially in girls (see Chapter 8). The intracranial lesions can arise *de novo* or be part of a predisposing condition such as neurofibromatosis (**4.13, 4.14**). Sexual precocity can also be seen rarely with primary long-standing hypothyroidism.

PSEUDO-SEXUAL PRECOCITY

This is characterized by:
- Hypertrophy of the target tissue of the hormone being secreted in excess.
- Regression or inhibition of the structures that usually secrete the hormone at puberty.
- Advanced bone maturation.
- Accelerated growth rate.

The development may be iso- or, less commonly, hetero-sexual and its causes include liver and adrenal tumors producing either testosterone or estrogen, non-salt-losing congenital virilizing adrenal hyperplasia (**4.15**) (see also Chapters 6 and 8), exogenous gonadotropin or sex steroid administration, gonadal tumors producing estrogen or testosterone, gonadotropin or human chorionic gonadotropin (hCG)-producing tumors and estrogen-secreting ovarian cysts (**4.16, 4.17**). Heterosexual pseudo-precocity in a female will often result in considerable clitoral hypertrophy (see Chapter 6) and this helps in the differentiation from premature adrenarche (see below).

Additionally, the McCune–Albright syndrome produces discordant sexual development. The syndrome consists of irregular pigmented café au lait patches, usually unilateral on the upper body (**1.127**). There are areas of bony dysplasia and cysts in the long bones (**4.18**) and skull (**4.19**). Pubertal signs are usually dis-

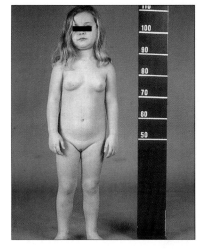

4.7 Central precocious puberty in female. Breasts stage 3, pubic hair stage 2, height 114 cm (3 ft 9 in) or +1.3SD at age 5.5 years

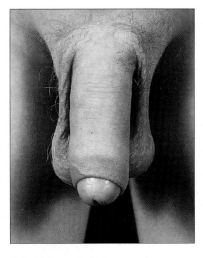

4.8 Male genitalia in central precocious puberty showing concordant pubertal development.

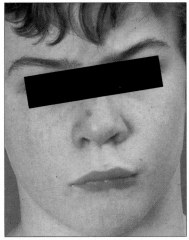

4.9 Early acne in male precocious puberty.

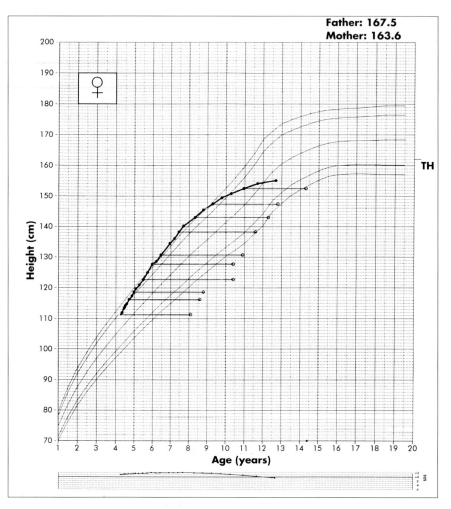

Father: 167.5
Mother: 163.6

4.10 Precocious puberty presenting at 4.3 years with a bone age of 8.2 years. Treatment with intra-nasal gonadotropin analog therapy delayed menarche to 11.5 years and subsequent bony fusion to around 12 years, but with evidence of a reduced final height of -1 SDS.

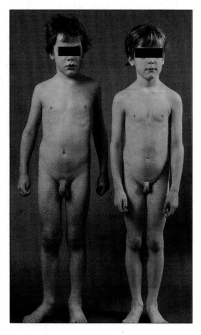

4.11 Male precocious puberty due to hamartoma, with unaffected twin brother.

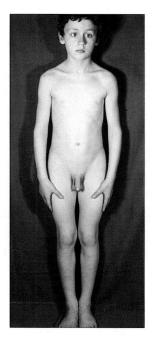

4.12 Male central precocious puberty with VIth nerve palsy secondary to intracranial astrocytoma.

cordant with early bleeding in females and no evidence of gonadotropin cyclicity. It is much more common in girls than boys and can also rarely cause thyrotoxicosis, gigantism and the Cushing syndrome. It appears to result from a generalized mutation of the G protein (a secondary messenger signaling receptor activation) in endocrine tissues, leading to overactivity.

Separately from the pathological secretion from tumors described above, excess production of estrogen from peripheral aromatase conversion of testosterone in an often overweight male can cause pubertal gynecomastia (**4.20**). Male breast development and lactorrhea from a prolactinoma is extremely uncommon. Testotoxicosis is a rare condition of familial male pseudo-precocious puberty leading to generally consonant changes of male puberty but with testes that are often small for the degree of virilization present (**4.21**, **4.22**). There is an absence of cyclical gonadotropin activation but a mutation causing a 'locking-on' of the testicular LH receptor is present, leading to early production of testosterone in the absence of circulating LH.

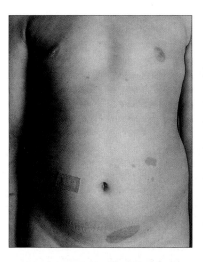

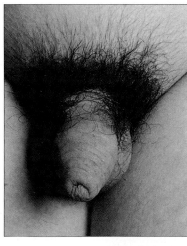

4.13, 4.14 Precocious puberty in neurofibromatosis. Note site of gonadotropin analog injection (with plaster), as well as the enlargement of testes and penis with consonant pubic hair growth. Secondary to optic glioma.

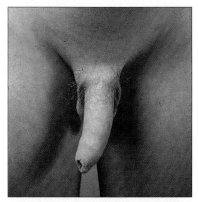

4.15 Non-salt losing 21-hydroxylase deficiency presenting late in a male with penile enlargement, pubic hair growth but small testes (indicating a non-testicular source of androgen).

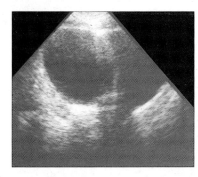

4.16 Large estrogen secreting ovarian cyst (on left of picture), pushing bladder and uterus to the right.

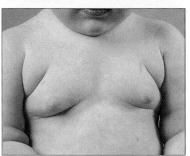

4.17 Premature breast development secondary to an ovarian cyst.

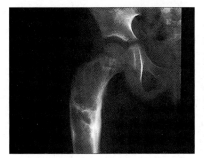

4.18 Fibrous dysplasia of upper femur.

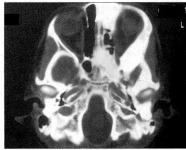

4.19 Fibrous dysplasia of base of skull and left orbit.

PREMATURE ADRENARCHE OR PUBARCHE

Characterized by:
- Pubic and axillary hair growth (**4.23, 1.101**).
- Acne, body odor and other androgen-mediated effects.
- A mildly advanced bone age.
- Usually no acceleration of height velocity.

The event termed 'adrenarche' is a normal age-related physiological maturation of the adrenal cortex, probably under the influence of ACTH (or another postulated 'central adrenarche stimulating hormone' CASH), producing increased secretion of dehydro-epiandrosterone (DHEA) and its sulphate (DHEAS) and other androgenic precursors of testosterone. Its effects are usually incorporated into puberty. If early maturation occurs then the mild virilizing effects become cosmetically noticeable. Idiopathic dislocation of adrenarche from puberty is commoner in girls than boys. Premature adrenarche can also be secondary to non-progressive intracranial lesions, presumably mediated by abnormal production of ACTH/CASH. The commonest intracranial causes are hydrocephalus and following meningitis, especially TB meningitis. It can occasionally be a familial event, in which case differentiation from late presenting atypical or non-classical congenital adrenal hyperplasia (see below) may be required.

HIRSUTISM

Other than adrenarche, excess hair production in the female (with or without later male-pattern baldness) can be due to other causes of excess adrenal activity or androgen production:
- Classical simple congenital adrenal hyperplasia.
- Late onset congenital adrenal hyperplasia is common but often undiagnosed. The non-classical sub-type is associated with human lymphocyte antigens (HLA) types B14 and B35 (see Chapter 6).
- The Cushing syndrome.
- Secondary to abnormal levels of testosterone produced by polycystic ovaries which can themselves be due to adrenal over-activity and hyperinsulinemia or occur as a primary event after puberty.
- Idiopathic hirsutism is possibly due to over activity of skin 5α-reductase levels. This can be treated with enzyme blockers such as finasteride.
- Some girls or their parents perceive cosmetic problems that are due only to normal growth of dark hair.

It is said that hirsutism confined to the lower body is indicative of an adrenal source of androgens.

As well as treating any identified underlying cause it is also appropriate to advise cosmetic treatments such as bleaching, depilation and electrolysis.

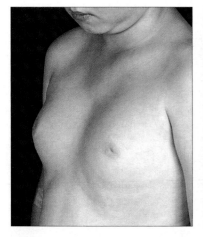

4.20 Gynecomastia, required surgical resection.

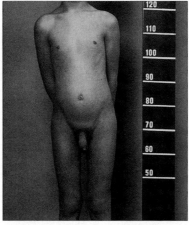

4.21 Testotoxicosis, there is stage 4 penis and pubic hair growth but only 6 ml testes.

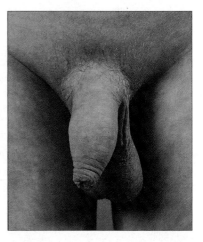

4.22 Genitalia in another case of testotoxicosis. More concordant development but a family history of the condition.

PREMATURE THELARCHE

This benign condition is characterized by:
- Early breast enlargement (**4.24**) usually in infancy, but which can occur throughout childhood and which is often cyclical over periods of months.
- The absence of the subsequent appearance of any other pubertal changes.
- Normal growth and skeletal maturation.

In premature thelarche waves of follicular development (above 3-4 mm) occur with FSH induction of aromatase. Low levels of estrogen can be detected by ultra-sensitive assays. A variant condition has been described with features intermediate between true central precocious puberty and thelarche.

DIAGNOSTIC WORK-UP

MEDICAL HISTORY AND PHYSICAL EXAMINATION

The following items are of importance in the history:
- The exact timing of the onset of pubertal signs, including in a girl whether breast development occurred earlier or later than pubic hair growth.
- Vaginal discharge, which may be creamy or blood-stained.
- Growth pattern. (Any rapid growth recently? This may be manifested by change relative to peers or changes in clothes and shoe size).

- Any symptoms suggestive of hypothyroidism?
- Any neurological or visual symptoms?
- Any family history of precocity or suggestive of neurofibromatosis?
- Previous diseases leading to neurological damage.
- Any exposure to drugs (estrogens, androgens, cimetidine)? This can be iatrogenic, accidental (e.g. ingestion of the contraceptive pill), or factitious. There are also reports of traditional Chinese herbal remedies leading to both male and female precocity.
- Dietary exposure to contaminated poultry or beef where excessive veterinary administration may be a possibility.

The physical examination should concentrate on:
- A precise description of pubertal stage. (For longitudinal follow-up it is useful to measure breast diameter.)
- Height, sitting height and weight and their evaluation versus age references and previous measurements. (As growth of the back is partly mediated by sex hormone secretion, early puberty will tend to produce a somewhat longer sitting height in relation to leg length.)
- Inspection of the color of the vulval mucosa. A pale color indicates estrogen activity (**4.25**).
- Signs of hyperandrogenization (hirsutism, clitoral or penile enlargement, acne). Hirsutism may be graded according to a simple scale (**4.26**).

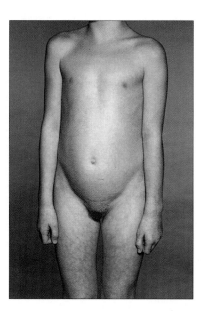

4.23 Premature adrenarche / pubarche. No breast development and stage 3 pubic hair growth. There was an adult body odor and mild acne but no cliteromegaly.

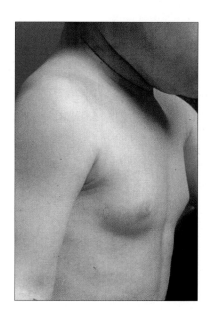

4.24 Premature thelarche.

- Blood pressure (elevated in the 11β-hydroxylase form of adrenal hyperplasia or with raised intracranial pressure).
- A search for pigmented birth marks.
- Thyroid size and signs of hypothyroidism (see Chapter 7). (In the male the testicular volume may be increased to a greater extent than might be expected from the other pubertal signs. In the female periods may occur earlier than would be expected for the stage of breast development.)
- Hepatomegaly or abdominal mass.
- Pelvic mass (e.g. ovarian cyst or tumor) on abdominal or rectal examination.
- Neurological examination (including fundoscopy).

INTERPRETATION OF THE CLUES

True precocity:
- In a girl with no other signs or symptoms = likely to be idiopathic (but check CT/MRI scan).
- With neurological signs or symptoms = central nervous system lesion.

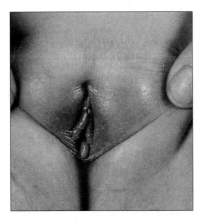

4.25 Genitalia of same case as shown in **4.16**, showing early maturation of vulval mucosa.

- With more than five café au lait spots and axillary freckles, with or without a positive family history = neurofibromatosis and optic glioma or other CNS tumor.
- Thyroid enlargement and/or typical symptoms and signs = hypothyroidism.

Pseudo-precocity:
- A positive family history = adrenarche or atypical 21-hydroxylase deficiency.
- Hypertension in a girl with virilization or in a boy with pseudo-precocious puberty = 11β-hydroxylase deficiency.
- Cliteromegaly plus advanced bone age and accelerated growth = androgenization not secondary to adrenarche.
- Irregular café au lait spots and/or lytic bone lesions on X-ray = McCune–Albright syndrome.
- Pelvic mass or mass felt per rectum = ovarian tumor.
- Hepatomegaly = hepatic tumor (producing sex hormones or hCG).
- Abdominal mass = adrenal tumor.
- Gynecomastia with unilateral testicular enlargement = germ cell tumor.
- Gynecomastia with no testicular enlargement = intra-abdominal tumor (often impalpable) or extra-glandular aromatase conversion at puberty (commonest in, but not exclusive to, obese subjects).
- Previous diseases leading to neurological damage = premature adrenarche.
- Early onset with cyclical breast enlargement = premature thelarche.
- Positive family history in a boy = familial testotoxicosis.

Simple grading of hirsutism				
Score	1	2	3	4
Lip	Few outer hairs	Outer margin	>50%	Full
Chin	Few hairs	Scattered	Light cover	Heavy
Lower abdomen	Few, midline	Midline streak	Band	Inverted 'V'
Thigh	Sparse, <25%	>25%	Complete, light	Heavy

Score each feature and add up the total. A score greater than 5 is indicative of significant hirsutism. The score can be used to document progression or regression of the signs.

4.26 Simple grading of hirsutism.

FURTHER INVESTIGATIONS

The evaluation of the growth pattern in the light of the pubertal stage is crucial for determining the number of further investigations. The sex of the child is also relevant.

Girls

If there is only a minor degree of breast enlargement in a young girl, with no other signs of estrogen activity and a normal growth pattern, further investigations can be limited to a hand and wrist radiograph for bone age. If bone age is not advanced, one could review the child after some months to see if the signs have subsided or progressed with pubic hair growth and also measure height velocity. If there is no progression of pubertal signs and a normal growth rate, the diagnosis is most likely to be premature thelarche or a temporary exposure to exogenous estrogens. Further review should be arranged and the carer instructed to return urgently if any more pubertal changes occur. A pelvic ultrasound examination that showed one or two follicles in a low-volume ovary with no sign of uterine enlargement would give further reassurance (**4.27**).

If there are definite signs of estrogen activity (active breast development, pale mucosa of introitus, psychological changes, growth acceleration, bone age acceleration), the following investigations are indicated:
- Basal estradiol (E_2), LH, FSH.
- Thyroid function tests: (F)T_4 and TSH.
- Abdominal ultrasound (ovarian and uterine size) (**4.28, 4.29**).

- In case of doubt about the estrogen results, vaginal cytology can be considered.
- GnRH test (see Appendix A) in a specialized center. Before puberty, the rise of LH and FSH is low, with usually a greater rise of FSH than of LH. During puberty, the increase of both gonadotropins is higher, with LH rising higher than FSH. Therefore, the ratio between LH and FSH (>1) can be used as a marker of 'real' puberty.

If there is positive evidence for true precocious puberty (E_2 > 50 pmol/L, LH / FSH ratio > 1, LH peak elevated) and no hypothyroidism, further investigations to find the precise cause are needed with an MRI or CT scan of the brain.

If there is positive evidence for pseudo-precocious puberty (elevated E_2, depressed LH and FSH levels even after GnRH) further investigations should be aimed at elucidating the precise cause. Sonography of the ovary, liver and adrenals should show the majority of tumors, although they can occasionally be intra-thoracic.

If there are mild signs of androgen excess and if growth and bone age are normal, the diagnosis is almost certainly benign precocious adrenarche and no further investigations are needed. (For documentation one can measure plasma DHEA and DHEAS, which are usually slightly elevated, and a urinary steroid profile which will show a mild elevation of adrenal cortical metabolites.) In non-classical 21-hydroxylase deficiency, which may mimic precocious adrenarche, a short ACTH test (see Appendix A) to provide an estimate of the basal levels and rise of 17α-hydroxyprogesterone may be required to prove the diagnosis.

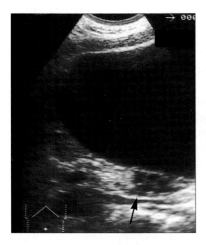

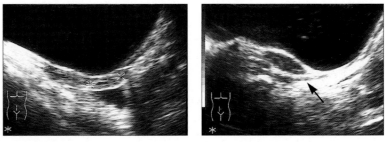

4.28, 4.29 Central precocious puberty demonstrated in girl presenting at 5 years with breast stage 2. There is enlargement of the uterus such that the body (+–+ 29 mm) is > cervix (x–x 19 mm). There is ovarian enlargement with the beginnings of peripheral follicle formation. This can occur only as part of cyclical gonadotropin secretion.

4.27 The ovaries in premature thelarche show a few large cysts/follicles in small volume glands. The uterus (not shown here) is of prepubertal size and shape.

If there is more severe virilization with cliteromegaly, accelerated height velocity and bone maturation then a urinary steroid profile and measurement of plasma or salivary 17α-hydroxyprogesterone, DHEA, DHEAS and androstenedione will allow the diagnosis of most forms of congenital adrenal hyperplasia and androgen-producing tumors. Tumors can be localized with ultrasound or CT scanning.

If there is abnormal pigmentation, X-rays of the skeleton will help confirm McCune–Albright syndrome, in which case thyroid and adrenal function should also be checked.

Boys

If there are definite signs of puberty with enlarging testes, basal serum testosterone, LH and FSH should be measured and a GnRH test performed in a specialist center. If testosterone is elevated (>1.0 nmol/l) and the GnRH test shows a pubertal pattern (see above), true precocious puberty is diagnosed. As the frequency of cerebral abnormalities in boys with true precocious puberty is relatively high, a CT or MRI scan is mandatory (**4.30, 4.31**).

If the testosterone is elevated, with small soft testes, pseudo-precocious puberty is likely and LH and FSH will remain suppressed during the GnRH test. Further determinations of other steroids in the urine and plasma (androstenedione, DHEAS, DHEA and 17α-hydroxyprogesterone) are indicated to determine the source of the androgens. It is possible to use the relative values to distinguish between premature adrenarche (relatively rare in the male), exogenous anabolic steroid administration, the various non-salt-losing forms of congenital adrenal hyperplasia and adrenal tumors.

If isolated gynecomastia is present then testosterone, prolactin, estrogen (E$_2$), hCG and LH levels should be measured. hCG and/or E$_2$ are elevated in some estrogen-secreting tumors that may be testicular (detected by ultrasonography), or extra-gonadal (detected by further ultrasonography or CT scanning). Primary testicular damage with elevated

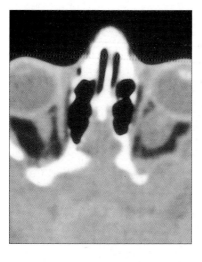
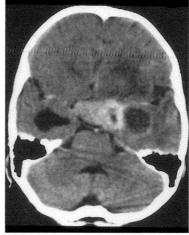

4.30, 4.31 Optic glioma producing sexual precocity in a male with neurofibromatosis. Thickened left optic nerve and chiasmatic tumor.

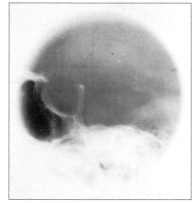

4.32 Massive enlargement of pituitary fossa secondary to prolactinoma.

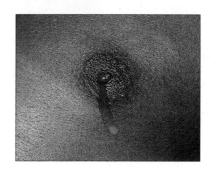

4.33 Lactorrhea.

menopausal LH levels (and hypothalamic or pituitary hypogonadism with undetectable LH levels) also may present with gynecomastia (obviously in the absence of other signs of sexual maturation, see Chapter 6). Prolactinomas in childhood (**4.32**) are extremely rare and usually present with CNS signs, although this is the only cause, if seen, of lactorrhea (**4.33**). If the estrogen is only slightly raised or all the tests are normal, then extra-glandular aromatase conversion of testosterone to estrogen is likely.

THERAPY

True precocious puberty will result in a reduced final height and early pubertal development can lead to psychological problems. For these reasons treatment is usually offered in specialist units. Current therapy uses depot slow-release GnRH-analogs intramuscularly or subcutaneously (depending on the preparation), every four weeks. Alternatively, short acting intra-nasal analogs can be used two or three times a day although the required strict compliance with this regime can be a problem.

To prevent initial hyperstimulation and worsening of the precocity it is usual to treat concurrently for the first six weeks with the oral sex-steroid synthesis blocker, cyproterone acetate (100 mg/m^2 body surface per 24 hours, divided into 2 or 3 doses). (Cyproterone acetate alone can be used as prolonged therapy for sexual precocity but, whilst effective in stopping the progress of pubertal development, it does not influence final height. It may be associated with side effects, like fatigue and liver dysfunction,

and biochemically it leads to hypocortisolism so that a stress regimen of glucocorticoids is necessary.)

Gonadotropin releasing hormone analog treatment is continued until the final height prediction has become acceptable and the child's peer group is showing pubertal changes. Puberty will then continue from the point of initiation of therapy and there are currently no long term recognized side effects.

Testotoxicosis and the McCune–Albright syndrome, both being gonadotropin independent, will not respond to GnRH analog treatment and hence cyproterone acetate or ketoconazole (which blocks several steps in adrenal steroid synthesis, including testosterone) is the most reasonable choice of therapy. Early central puberty may supervene and additional GnRH treatment may be necessary.

Pseudo-precocity secondary to tumorous sources of sex steroids requires expert oncological and surgical intervention. Any of the forms of congenital adrenal hyperplasia presenting with virilization (with or without hypertension) are treated with steroid replacement as should late presenting non-classical 21-hydroxylase deficiency (see Chapters 6 and 8).

Adrenarche is benign, though of cosmetic importance, as is isolated hirsutism. Excess hair can be treated with depilatory creams and electrolysis. Acne can be ameliorated by skin cleansers and topical antibiotic preparations. In the older patient anti-androgens combined with a contraceptive preparation could be considered under careful supervision. Thelarche requires no intervention.

Idiopathic gynecomastia is best treated by an experienced plastic surgeon as the results of medical therapy are disappointing.

5.

Late Sexual Development

A delay or lack of pubertal development is diagnosed if breast stage 2 in girls has not started at 13–14 years of age and if genital stage 2 (testicular volume ≥4 ml) has not started in boys at 15–16 years of age. Because of the lack of a pubertal growth spurt many of these patients will present primarily with short stature (see Chapter 2).

CLASSIFICATION OF LATE PUBERTY

Delayed puberty is classified according to the serum gonadotropin levels: high gonadotropin concentrations indicate primary gonadal failure and low gonadotropin concentrations indicate disorders at the hypothalamic-pituitary level.

HYPERGONADOTROPIC HYPOGONADISM

Congenital primary gonadal failure is associated with:
- Gonadal dysgenesis associated with sex chromosome abnormalities (the Ullrich–Turner syndrome, Klinefelter syndrome, etc.).
- Idiopathic syndromic abnormalities. There are more than twenty named syndromes which are associated with hypergonadotropic hypogonadism.
- Genetic disorders of enzyme production causing sex steroid deficiency.
- Pure gonadal dysgenesis (defective germ cell migration).
- Complete androgen insensitivity caused by receptor/post-receptor abnormalities. Here the gonads are functional but the tissues unresponsive (see Chapter 6). Complete forms that do not present as female infants with bilateral inguinal hernias usually present as primary amenorrhea.

Acquired primary gonadal failure is associated with:
- Autoimmune disorders.
- Galactosemia.
- Infections.
- Irradiation to the gonad and some chemotherapy regimes (see Chapter 8).
- Trauma, *in utero* or later torsion, 'vanishing testes' etc.

HYPOGONADOTROPIC HYPOGONADISM

Temporary deficiency, associated with delayed maturation, can result from:
- Constitutional delay of growth and adolescence (physiological).
- Chronic illnesses and systemic diseases.
- Hypothyroidism (also associated with sexual precocity).
- Anorexia nervosa.
- Excessive physical training.
- Excessive emotional and/or physical stress.
- Malnutrition.

Permanent pathological deficiency may be:
- Isolated (with anosmia = Kallmann syndrome).
- Part of a syndromic malformation. (Again there are a number of eponymous conditions associated with central gonadotropin lack.)
- In the context of multiple pituitary deficiencies, idiopathic or due to anatomical malformations and acquired lesions.

DIAGNOSTIC WORK-UP

MEDICAL HISTORY AND EXAMINATION

Features of importance in the history include:
- Family history of delayed sexual development.
- Family history of autoimmune or endocrine disease.
- Parental size.
- Birth and pregnancy details.
- Any learning problems?
- Previous medical treatments and surgery, including 'minor' procedures such as orchidopexy or neonatal hernia repair.
- Disordered eating behavior.
- Sense of smell absent. (A patient with anosmia may be able to detect the presence of an odor, especially of volatile substances, but be unable to differentiate between smells.)
- Social pressures, the sexual development of the close peer group.
- Levels of exercise.

The physical examination should concentrate on:

- Height (see **2.1**), weight, adiposity.
- Body proportions. (As much of the growth of the back at puberty is mediated by sex hormone secretion, patients with delayed puberty, but no other endocrinopathy, will tend to have long legs compared to their backs, the so-called eunuchoid body proportions (**5.1**).)
- Hirsutism (see Chapter 4).
- Lanugo hair (may be a sign of eating disorders) (**5.2**).
- Hernia repairs or other operative scars.
- External genital appearance (measure gently stretched penis length, see Chapter 6). Anatomical abnormalities of the genital tract such as imperforate hymen, absent uterus etc, presenting as primary amenorrhea without delay of other sexual characteristics, may require ultrasonic investigation, examination under anesthesia or laparoscopy.
- The presence of cryptorchidism (**5.3**).
- Dysmorphic features.
- Signs of thyroid disease.
- Neurological signs.
- Gynecomastia (see **4.20**).
- Lactorrhea (see **4.32**, **4.33**).
- Testing sense of smell.

INTERPRETATION OF THE CLUES

- Typical dysmorphic features and short stature = the Ullrich–Turner syndrome (see Chapter 2). Remember that up to 40% of girls with the Ullrich–Turner syndrome will have no external phenotypic abnormality (**5.4–5.6**).
- Dysmorphic features, short stature and obesity = Prader–Labhart–Willi syndrome (**5.7, 5.8**).
- Dysmorphic features, other abnormalities such as retinitis pigmentosa (see **1.111**) = syndromic malformation such as the Bardet–Biedl or Laurence–Moon syndrome.
- Other specific dysmorphic syndromes and hypogonadism.
- Tall stature, disproportion and cryptorchidism or small firm testes = Klinefelter syndrome.
- Under-virilized male with gynecomastia and hypertension = late presenting 17α-hydroxylase deficiency.
- Under-virilized male or phenotypic 46XY female with late virilization = late presenting partial 17-ketosteroid reductase deficiency (or 17β-hydroxysteroid dehydrogenase deficiency); partial androgen insensitivity syndrome (see Chapter 6).

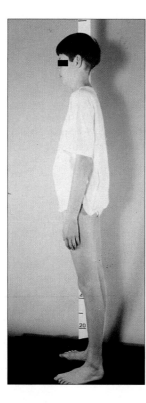

5.1 Eunuchoid body habitus (47 XXY).

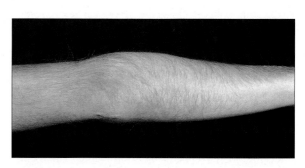

5.2 Excess lanugo hair.

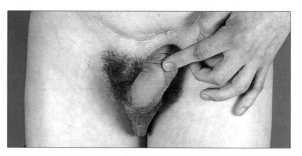

5.3 Cryptorchidism, here with functioning intra-abdominal testes.

- Failure of breast development, often with some evidence of adrenal androgen activity = gonadal dysgenesis (**5.9**).
- Hypogonadism with alopecia, vitiligo, candidiasis = autoimmune polyendocrinopathy 3c (**5.10**).
- Family history of delay (often in same sex parent or sib) = constitutional delay of growth and adolescence.
- Extreme thinness or falling weight, disordered eating and behavior in relation to food = anorexia nervosa (**5.11**). Past anorexia can cause severe

delay of puberty for many years after successful restoration of adequate weight (**5.12**). In addition to this psychiatric spectrum simple fear of obesity with dieting is very common and can produce delay.
- Anosmia, small penis and testes or cryptorchidism = Kallmann syndrome.
- Hypogonadism and lactorrhea = prolactinoma (**4.32–4.33**).
- Hypogonadism with hypothyroidism and short stature = panhypopituitarism (**5.13**, **5.14**).

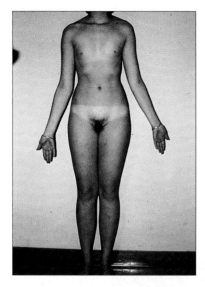

5.4 Ullrich–Turner syndrome with few dysmorphic features except infantilism and a wide carrying angle.

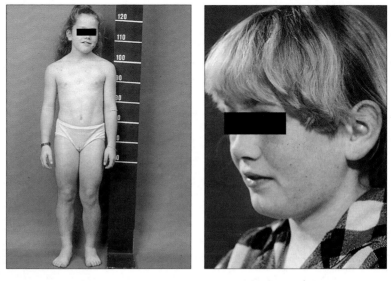

5.5, 5.6 Two cases of Ullrich–Turner syndrome with no dysmorphic features.

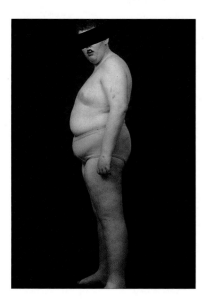

5.7 Prader–Labhart–Willi syndrome.

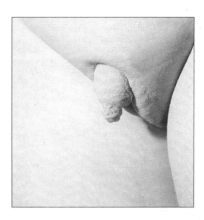

5.8 Close-up of genitalia in Prader–Labhart–Willi syndrome.

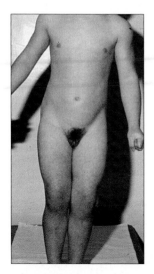

5.9 Gonadal dysgenesis with adrenal source of pubic hair.

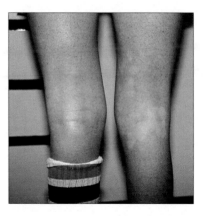

5.10 Vitiligo.

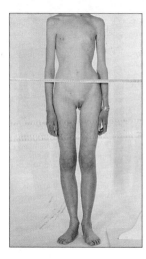

5.11 Anorexia nervosa.

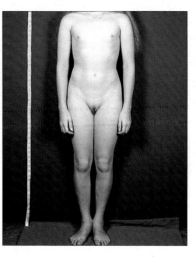

5.12 Past anorexia causing later extreme delay of puberty (menses at 20 years).

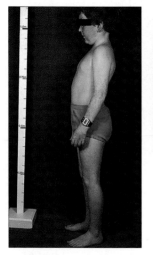

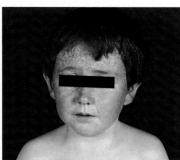

5.13, 5.14 Panhypopituitarism with infantilism, age 13.5 years (whole body view and facial close-up).

FURTHER INVESTIGATIONS

On the basis of a proper history and physical examination, a tentative diagnosis can often be made. Thereafter, basal serum testosterone or estradiol and gonadotropins should be performed in specialized units along with a bone age. In permanent hyper- or hypogonadotropic hypogonadism bone age can be higher than 11 (girls) or 13 (boys) years in the absence of pubertal signs, while this is unusual in temporary deficiency. Thereafter tests will depend on whether there is hyper- or hypogonadotropism.

Hypergonadotropic hypogonadism
By definition the gonadotropins are elevated, and often the FSH to a greater extent than the LH.

Even in the absence of abnormal genitalia or dysmorphic features, a karyotype should be performed. It may be necessary to take both blood and fibroblast specimens to exclude tissue mosaicism.

If there is hypertension, a urinary adrenal steroid profile will help diagnose variants of steroid synthesis disorders.

Pelvic ultrasonography will reveal absence of even small prepubertal ovaries if streak gonads are present. In a male with impalpable testes they may be localised with ultrasonography either in the inguinal canal or intra-abdominally. To determine if there is functioning gonadal tissue, a short hCG (human chorionic gonadotropin) test can be performed (see Appendix A). Administration of this LH-like compound will cause production of estrogen or testosterone that can be measured as a rise from the basal values. Occasionally a prolonged test is required for absolute proof of lack of gonadal tissue.

In a male with impalpable gonads and a rise in testosterone in response to hCG, but in whom ultrasonography fails to localize the tissue, laparoscopy is needed to assess the possibility of orchidopexy or the need for gonadectomy to prevent undetected malignant change.

Auto-antibodies to the thyroid, adrenal and ovary can be estimated in the presence of a family history or suggestive physical signs.

Hypogonadotropic hypogonadism
To differentiate between permanent and temporary gonadotropin deficiency, a GnRH test can be performed (see Appendix A). The results may be equivocal as, although complete failure of a rise of gonadotropin concentration is suggestive of central hypogonadism, a blunted response can occur just prior to the onset of delayed puberty. Differentiation from partial central deficiency may thus be difficult without serial re-testing before or after a period of treatment, (see below.)

If there is short stature or signs of hypothyroidism then a combined anterior pituitary function test with basal thyroid function (FT4) is indicated (see Appendix A), along with imaging of the central nervous system if multiple deficiencies are proven.

Occasionally, the short stature and long legs (in comparison to the back) that is seen in delayed puberty can be mimicked by the milder forms of spondyloepiphyseal dysplasia and a limited skeletal survey may be needed.

THERAPY

Hypergonadotropic hypogonadism
In males, counseling is indicated about the need for treatment (long-term testosterone), infertility, and the option of testicular prostheses. Testosterone treatment is started at about 12 years (50–100 mg once a month by depot i.m. injection or oral testosterone undecanoate, 40 mg alternate days increasing to a daily dose after 6 months) to ensure a normal physical and psychosocial development, normal sexual function and to protect the cardiovascular system and bone mineral density. Testicular prostheses are usually placed at the end of pubertal development and the dose of testosterone increased (250 mg by depot i.m. injection once every three weeks or oral testosterone undecanoate 80–240 mg per day), to achieve a normal level of sexual activity.

In females treatment is needed with estrogens to induce breast development, to prevent osteoporosis and to ensure a normal psychosocial development. Ethinylestradiol is commonly used. The starting dosage is 0.05 µg per kg body weight given orally (usually about 2 µg per day or alternate days). An initial low dosage appears to improve final height by preventing early bony fusion and there is an improved cosmetic appearance of the breasts. The dosage is gradually increased over a period of two or three years to reach a substitution dosage of 20–30 µg with progestagens at a dosage of 5–10 mg medroxyprogesterone per day for 10–14 days per month. When growth is completed, trans-cutaneous patches or a triphasic contraceptive pill can be conveniently used. Counseling about infertility is required although the use of egg donation and gametocyte transfer allows the possible artificial induction of pregnancy in some individuals.

Hypogonadotropic hypogonadism
Initially in males it may be difficult to separate constitutional delay from central hypogonadism. For psychological reasons a pragmatic approach is to offer testosterone treatment. This may be given either in a depot dosage of 50–100 mg of testosterone esters every 3–4 weeks intra-muscularly or

as oral testosterone undecanoate 20–40 mg per day. An alternative approach is to use the anabolic steroid oxandrolone in a dose of 1.25–2.5 mg per day orally. Usually these treatments are discontinued after three or four months and the development of testicular size is checked along with serum testosterone measurements. If puberty starts (testicular volume $\geqslant 4$ ml), testosterone /oxandrolone treatment can be stopped to allow natural puberty to progress. If there is failure of subsequent development a further three month course and re-evaluation of the possibility of permanent central hypogonadism may be necessary. In cases of a permanent gonadotropin deficiency, testosterone treatment is continued for life. Intermittent biosynthetic gonadotropin administration, hMG (human menopausal gonadotropin), hCG and pulsatile GnRH infusion have all been used to induce spermatogenesis. Pure recombinant gonadotropins will soon become more generally available

In females, pubertal delay requiring treatment is rare but may be treated with low dosages of ethinylestradiol. In case of permanent central hypogonadism, estrogen substitution is indicated. The dosage is gradually increased over two to three years, for example from 4 to 10 to 20 and later 30 μg ethinylestradiol per day, while medroxyprogesterone is added to ensure regular menses (10–14 days per month). Patches or triphasic contraceptive preparations may again be used conveniently till menopausal age or hormone replacement therapy continued life-long.

Hypopituitary females often have sparse pubic hair growth (secondary to lack of adrenal maturation and androgen production). This cosmetic problem can be treated with topical or low dose oral / injected testosterone, or oral DHAS, if required.

6.

Abnormal Genitalia

NORMAL DEVELOPMENT OF THE GENITALIA

For the purpose of this book only a few aspects of genital development will be highlighted to facilitate understanding of the various disorders.

A crucial point is that the external genitalia develop 'automatically' in the female direction *unless* there is testosterone activity in a critical period between 4 and 12 weeks of gestation. Furthermore, the Müllerian ducts develop into the uterus and fallopian tubes *unless* Müllerian inhibiting factor (MIF) is produced and effective. Both hormones are produced only by the testis. Therefore the testis and the two hormones it produces are essential for the development of the genitalia, while the ovary and estrogens do not appear essential in that period.

The regulating process can be divided into various steps as shown in **6.1**. The first step is that the presence of one gene, called the testis determining gene (TDG), which usually resides on the Y chromosome, leads to the development of the undifferentiated gonad into a testis. Therefore, disorders at the chromosomal level can prevent the testis from differentiating. These disorders include mosaicisms of the sex chromosomes (e.g. 46XY/45X in mixed gonadal dysgenesis and many others), translocation of the TDG to another chromosome, e.g. an X-chromosome (XX-males **6.2**), and deletion of the TDG (XY-female). At a more subtle scale, abnormalities of the TDG (deletions, mutations) also lead to insufficient differentiation of the testis (XY females with gonadal dysgenesis). Chromosomal disorders (which can be generalized, chimeric or localized to the gonads) can

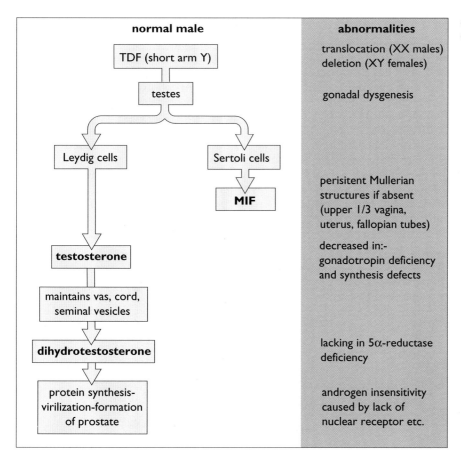

6.1 The process of genital development.

lead to an undifferentiated gonad or a dysgenetic testis or a combination of testicular and ovarian tissue as in true hermaphroditism.

After differentiation the normal testis produces testosterone and MIF. The presence of MIF leads to regression of the Müllerian ducts. If MIF production does not occur in the presence of a normal testosterone secretion, for example due to agenesis of Sertoli cells or a mutation in the MIF gene, the Müllerian duct develops into a uterus while the external genitalia are those of a normal male (**6.3**). As would be expected, MIF receptor abnormalities lead to a similar persistent Müllerian duct syndrome as is seen in MIF gene mutations or deletions.

The presence of testosterone normally leads to male differentiation of the external genitalia and development of the Wolffian ducts. If testosterone production does not occur, the external genitalia do not develop in the male direction and the Wolffian duct does not develop into the internal male duct (vas deferens). Lack of testosterone production may be due to agenesis of the Leydig cells, an inability of Leydig cells to produce testosterone (enzyme deficiencies of testosterone biosynthesis which are common to the testis and adrenal gland) or a lack of stimulation of testosterone secretion by insufficient production or action of placental hCG and pituitary gonadotropins.

Although directly active on embryonic Wolffian structures and muscle, testosterone can exert its effect on the external genitalia only if it is converted to dihydrotestosterone (DHT) within the target cells by 5α-reductase. DHT is subsequently bound to an androgen receptor and acts on the nucleus to exert its effects on the synthesis of virilizing proteins. Therefore, even if testosterone is produced normally, there can be disorders at the enzymatic, receptor and post-receptor level causing complete or partial insensitivity to the hormone. For instance, if the converting enzyme (5α-reductase) is absent or mutated, if the androgen receptor is absent or mutated or if

there are post-receptor disorders, the external genitalia will be either completely female or masculinized to an extent determined by the completeness of the defect – complete or partial androgen insensitivity syndrome (formerly called testicular feminization).

The commonest cause of excessive testosterone production leading to virilization in the female is congenital adrenal hyperplasia. Cortisol secretion is regulated in a classical feedback loop with ACTH and hence if cortisol secretion is blocked by any enzymatic deficiency in the adrenal, there is no negative feed-back, and increased ACTH secretion leads to an enlargement of the adrenal and over-secretion of steroid precursors and steroids not on the affected pathway (**6.4, 6.5**).

Of all the possible adrenal enzyme deficiencies, 21-hydroxylase deficiency is by far the most frequent with an incidence of between 1 in 5×10^3 and 1 in 20×10^3 births, depending on the population. There are two clinical variants of the 'classic' condition: the simple virilizing form, and the salt-wasting form. (There is also a late-onset 'non-classical' sub-type with less prominent clinical features.) Copies of the gene are carried on chromosome 6p and are closely linked to the HLA type of the individual. The defect is expressed only in the zona fasciculata in the simple virilizing form and in both the fasciculata and glomerulosa in the salt-wasting form. The salt-wasting form is strongly associated with HLA types BW47 and DR7. Similar variation in the expression of salt loss or the balance of over- or under-virilization seen, for instance, in 3ß hydroxysteroid dehydrogenase deficiency is presumably explained in a similar fashion.

The mechanism of synthesis of testosterone is the same in the adrenal and the testes. Enzyme deficiencies on this pathway leading to cortisol deficiency will thus lead to male pseudohermaphroditism with adrenal hyperplasia. Those defects 'lower down' the pathway (after 17, 20 desmolase) will have no effect on cortisol production and present with simple under-virilization.

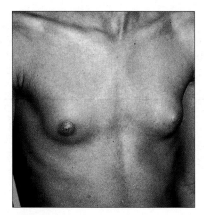

6.2 XX male presenting at puberty with gynecomastia.

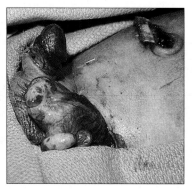

6.3 MIF deficiency. The uterus and fallopian tubes can be seen externalized at operation in this phenotypic male; penis visible top left.

GENDER IDENTITY

Any individual, whatever the disturbance in the process of genital differentiation, develops a gender identity, i.e. feels himself or herself a male or female. This gender identity is mostly based on the physical appearance of the external genitalia. This determines the behavior of the parents, and later of the child itself. A schematic picture of the development of gender identity is shown in **6.6**.

In cases in which the physical appearance of the external genitalia is ambiguous, a decision about the sex of rearing has to be made by the pediatrician, after establishing the diagnosis and weighing the long-term consequences of both options in conjunction with the carers. For this decision the likelihood of testosterone responsiveness and the size of the phallus are of paramount importance. In general, if there is evidence of resistance to testosterone and if the phallus is small, the child should be reared as a female, whatever the chromosomal or gonadal situation, because a normal male phallus is very difficult to create surgically. In such cases the physician must make very clear to the carers that such a child *is* female, rather than is being *made* female.

The severely masculinized XX individual with, for instance, congenital adrenal hyperplasia, has a good prognosis, with appropriate medical and surgical treatment, for sexual function and fertility when raised as a female. Clitoral reduction and later vaginoplasty can produce acceptable appearance and function.

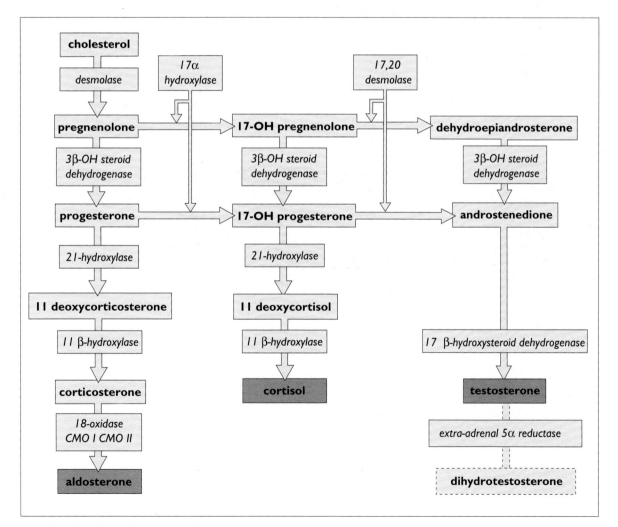

6.4 The adrenal steroid synthesis pathway.

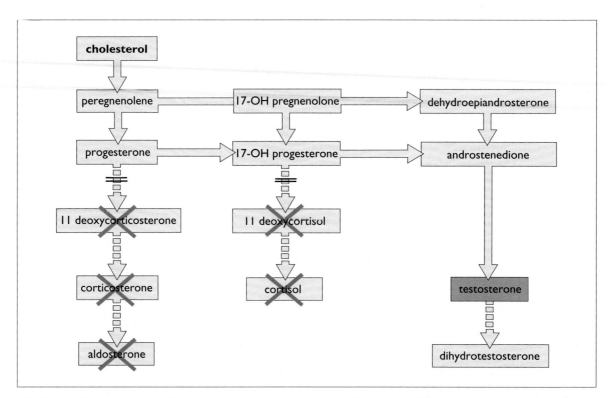

6.5 Schematic representation of the common form of congenital adrenal hyperplasia, 21-hydroxylase deficiency.

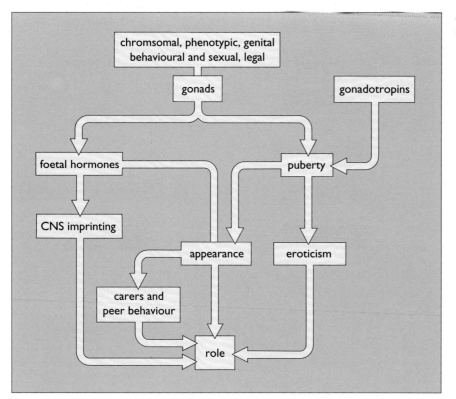

6.6 The components of sexual identity.

CLASSIFICATION

There are four groups of intersex disorders based on the appearance of the gonads.

1. Undifferentiated or absent gonads
Also known as abnormal gonadogenesis, with or without chromosomal abnormalities. There is some confusion about the classification if gonadal dysgenesis is associated with an XY chromosomal pattern; some authors classify these forms in the group of male pseudo-hermaphroditism and others in the group of undifferentiated gonads. In the present classification only the gross abnormalities of the gonads (XY pure gonadal dysgenesis, congenital anorchia [vanishing testes]) are included in this group.

2. True hermaphroditism
Characterized by the presence of both ovarian and testicular tissue (**6.7, 6.8**). Any pattern of sex chromosomes can be found in these cases.

3. Male pseudo-hermaphroditism
Characterized by insufficient masculinization in the presence of a testis. This can be sub-classified:
- Insufficient stimulation by gonadotropins: hypopituitarism (**6.9**) or isolated gonadotropin deficiency (**6.10**) which may be part of a syndrome (**6.11**); gonadotropin insensitivity; delayed hCG or LH receptor development. These defects more commonly present with isolated micropenis, but testicular development can sometimes be so poor that incomplete virilization occurs.

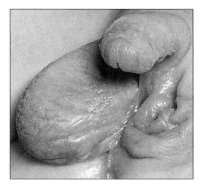

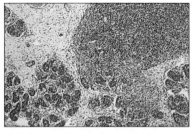

6.8 Histology of gonad in true hermaphroditism showing ovotestis. Ovarian tissue is shown as dense stroma with oocytes, testicular tissue shows tubule formation. Peripheral blood karyotype 100% normal 46XX, skin and gonadal tissue type chimeric 46XX/69XXY

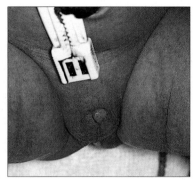

6.7 True hermaphrodite. Right sided descended testis, internal left ovo-testis, hypospadias.

6.9 Micropenis and cryptorchidism in panhypopituitarism. Infant had cleft palate and developed hypoglycemia.

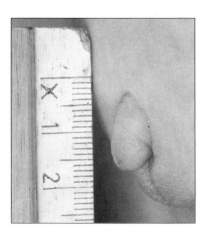

6.10 Micropenis and cryptorchidism in isolated gonadotropin deficiency.

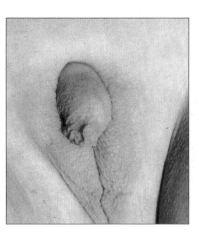

6.11 Micropenis and cryptorchidism in Prader–Labhart–Willi syndrome.

- Leydig cell agenesis.
- Disturbed androgen synthesis, because of enzymatic disorders: 20,22-desmolase also called congenital lipoid hyperplasia (**6.12, 6.13**), 17α-hydroxylase, 3β-hydroxysteroid dehydrogenase (**6.14**), 17,20-desmolase, 17-ketosteroid reductase (also called 17β-hydroxysteroid dehydrogenase deficiency) (**6.15–6.19**).
- Reduced 5α-reductase activity.
- Androgen insensitivity syndrome (AIS), complete or partial: androgen receptor or post receptor defect (**6.20–6.22**).
- Timing defect (late hormonal secretion *in utero*).
- Isolated MIF deficiency.
- Maternal ingestion of anti-androgens.
- Idiopathic.

4. Female pseudo-hermaphroditism

Characterized by excessive masculinization in the presence of ovaries. This is by far the commonest cause of abnormal genitalia. It may be sub-classified as:

- Congenital adrenal hyperplasia; 21-hydroxylase, accounting for 90% of all intersex; 11β-hydroxylase (about 5%) or 3β-hydroxysteroid dehydrogenase deficiency (about 1%).
- Excess of maternal androgens as either ingestion of androgens (or 19-nortestosterone derived progestagens) or virilizing tumors, luteomas and maternal congenital adrenal hyperplasia.
- Non-specific, associated with other congenital anomalies.
- Idiopathic (**6.23**).

Additionally, isolated **micropenis** and **cryptorchidism** will be considered in this chapter.

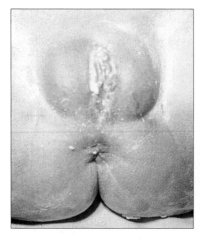

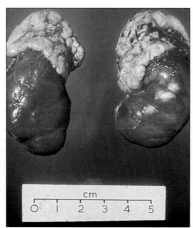

6.12, 6.13 Congenital lipoid hyperplasia, external appearance and post-mortem appearance of adrenals.

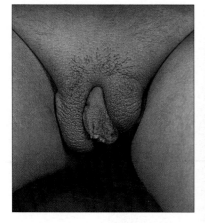

6.14 Non-salt losing 3β-hydroxysteroid dehydrogenase deficiency.

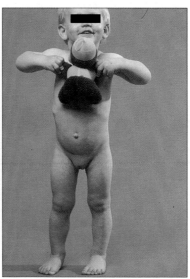

6.15 Karyotypic male with 17-ketosteroid reductase deficiency (17β-hydroxysteroid dehydrogenase deficiency).

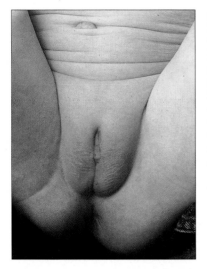

6.16–6.19
Karyotypic males with 17-ketosteroid reductase deficiency (17β-hydroxysteroid dehydrogenase deficiency), close-up of genital appearance to show variability. Note pigmentation in **6.17**.

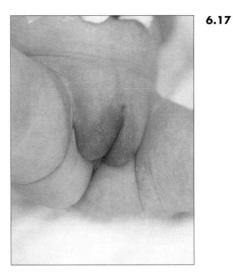

6.17

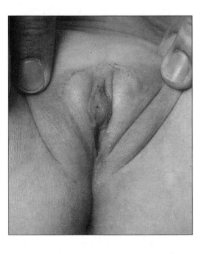

6.18

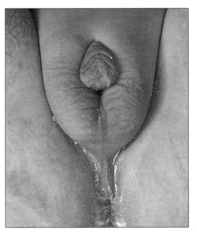

6.19

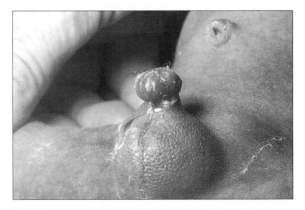

6.20 Partial androgen insensitivity with descended testes in bifid labio-scrotal folds.

6.21 Less severe partial androgen insensitivity with severe hypospadias and maldescent of testes.

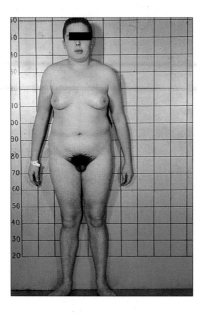

6.22 Partial androgen insensitivity syndrome, male sex of rearing, at adolescence. Note gynecomastia from peripheral aromatase conversion of testosterone to estrogen.

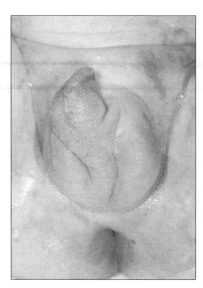

6.23 Masculinization of female infant. No cause found.

DIAGNOSTIC WORK-UP OF INTERSEX

HISTORY AND CLINICAL EXAMINATION

As with most congenital defects the history should concentrate on maternal health, pregnancy details and family history:
- Symptoms of virilization in the mother.
- Drugs during pregnancy.
- Unexplained infant deaths.
- Genital ambiguity, short stature or pronounced hirsutism in the family.
- Parental consanguinity.

The physical examination should include a thorough inspection and palpation of the external genitalia, blood pressure (elevated in 11β-hydroxylase deficiency) and a search for other congenital anomalies. Ambiguous genitalia include the whole spectrum from the normal male to normal female genitalia. Five intermediate stages have been distinguished by Prader (**6.24–6.30**). Any abnormality of the external genitalia should lead to further investigations including apparently normal female genitalia with palpable gonads in the labia or inguinal area, females with bilateral inguinal hernias or apparently normal males with impalpable gonads. (Male infants with congenital adrenal hyperplasia may show signs of excess testosterone production by an increase in scrotal pigmentation and a slight increase in penis size (**6.31, 6.32.**). These signs are often missed, however, and then the presentation is as collapse with hyponatremia and acidosis or, in non-salt losers, as the 'infantile Hercules syndrome' (see Chapter 8).

In cases of female pseudo-hermaphroditism the mother should be examined for signs of virilization and hypertension that would indicate a maternal source of testosterone.

INTERPRETATION OF THE CLUES

If gonads are palpable externally, there is at least a TDF present, usually on a Y chromosome. (In complete androgen insensitivity syndrome a proportion of cases will present with apparently normal female external genitalia but bilateral hernias, which contain testes.) Otherwise, in the absence of obvious maternal pathology or family history it is not wise to try to base a diagnosis on external appearance alone. Further elucidation will come from investigation in specialist centers.

INVESTIGATIONS

Karyotype
Many laboratories can provide a result, at least on the presence or absence of a Y chromosome, within a few days. The final result of the karyotype may take several weeks. (Buccal smears can be taken and investigated for the presence of Barr bodies. If seen, at least two X chromosomes are present. This investigation should be abandoned if rapid chromosome testing is available.) Chimerism can result in a normal peripheral kayotype with the abnormal chromosomes only expressed in gonadal tissue or skin. Further investigations are determined by the karyotype:

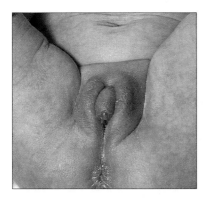

6.24

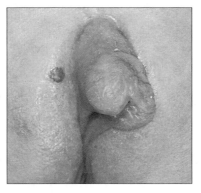

6.25

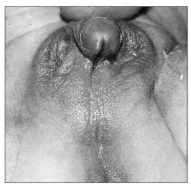

6.26

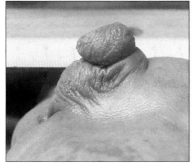

6.27

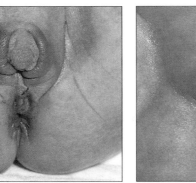

6.28

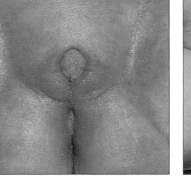

6.29

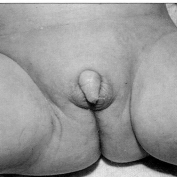

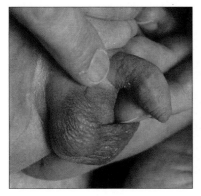

6.30

6.24–6.30 Stages of masculinization in 21-hydroxylase deficiency from relatively minor to complete in a series of karotypic females.
6.24 = Prader stage 1
6.25 = Prader stage 2
6.26 = Prader stage 3
6.27 = Prader stage 3
6.28 = Prader stage 4
6.29 = Prader stage 5
6.30 = External normal phenotypic male, 46XX

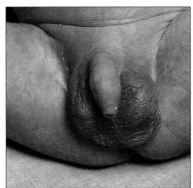

6.31, 6.32 Male genitalia in 21-hydroxylase deficiency, 46 XY.

XX karyotype

- Biochemical assessment should include several estimations of serum sodium and potassium. Some forms of congenital adrenal hyperplasia can lead to salt loss which is not always present in the first weeks.
- Kidney function should be checked, to detect any associated renal disorders. If these are suspected, in addition to ultrasonography, a renogram or intravenous pyelogram (IVP) should be obtained.
- The anatomy of the internal genitalia is investigated by ultrasonography (to check for gonads, uterus and vagina) and a contrast examination of the urogenital sinus. A cervical imprint seen with a contrast examination proves the presence of a uterus (**6.33**) that may not be apparent on ultrasound.
- Cystoscopy may be performed to evaluate the urethra and bladder.
- Laparoscopy may allow for the further differentiation of internal anatomy and direct visualization of the gonads along with possible gonadal biopsy.
- Plasma 17α-hydroxyprogesterone is raised in the commonest form of congenital adrenal hyperplasia, 21-hydroxylase deficiency (**6.4**). Additionally testosterone, androstenedione and dehydroepiandrosterone (DHEA and DHEAS) will be elevated and are responsible for the virilization that occurs. Cortisol production will be diminished and in 80% of cases there will be salt-losing, secondary to aldosterone deficiency.
- In 11ß-hydroxylase deficiency, plasma deoxycorticosterone -11 (DOC) and deoxycortisol will be elevated in addition to the above androgens (and there will be hypertension due to the salt retaining properties of DOC). Cortisol production will be diminished.
- In 3β-hydroxysteroid dehydrogenase deficiency there will be salt-losing and cortisol deficiency with elevated dehydroepiandrosterone (DHEA and DHEAS). Pregnenolone will be elevated and a urinary steroid profile will show a characteristic elevation of pregnenediol and pregnenetriol concentrations. This deficiency can cause both male and female pseudo-hermaphroditism, presumably depending on the activity of accessory pathways of testosterone synthesis from DHEA and DHEAS.
- Occasionally a urinary steroid profile, plasma steroid levels, ultrasonography and radiography will have to be performed on the mother to determine the source of androgens in an infant virilized secondary to a maternal cause.

XY karyotype

- Measurements of serum testosterone, dihydrotestosterone (DHT) and its steroid precursors, androstenedione and dehydroepiandrosterone (DHEA and DHEAS), should be performed, both before and after one hCG injection of 1500 IU, (see Appendix A). A normal testosterone rise excludes Leydig cell agenesis and enzymatic disorders of testosterone biosynthesis, and is more compatible with a partial androgen insensitivity syndrome, as the complete syndrome will have phenotypically normal female genitalia (**6.34**). The ratio between testosterone and its precursors indicates the precise level of enzyme defect in disorders of testosterone biosynthesis (**6.4**). A high ratio between androstenedione and testosterone indicates 17β-hydroxysteroid dehydrogenase deficiency; a high dehydroepiandrosterone indicates 3β-hydroxysteroid dehydrogenase defect; very low levels of 17α-hydroxyprogesterone, androstenedione and testosterone in the presence of high progesterone levels indicates 17α-hydroxylase deficiency; high progesterone and 17α-hydroxyprogesterone levels with low androstenedione and testosterone levels

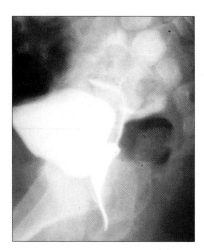

6.33 Cloacagram showing filling of vagina, fistula to bladder, cervical imprint and uterine cavity.

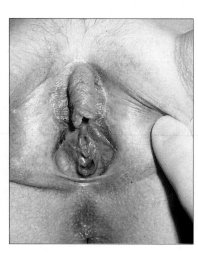

6.34 Complete androgen insensitivity syndrome presenting at puberty with sparse pubic hair growth and amenorrhea.

indicate a 17,20-desmolase deficiency. Very low levels of all steroids are seen in Leydig cell aplasia and if the first set of enzymes converting cholesterol to pregnenolone (desmolase) is deficient. If testosterone increases and there is little or no rise in DHT then the defect lies in the conversion of testosterone to DHT by 5α-reductase.

- The sex hormone binding globulin (SHBG) response to the anabolic steroid stanazolol can be used to estimate the degree of androgen insensitivity. Unfortunately the test is reliable only after four months of age. In normal individuals there is a 50% reduction in SHBG from the baseline, four days after a three day course of treatment with 0.5 mg/kg. In complete AIS there is no response or even a slight rise in levels. Those with a fall of less than 20% will probably not respond sufficiently to later treatment to be successfully raised as males.
- Genital skin fibroblasts can be obtained for assay of androgen receptor levels and elucidation of post-receptor defects in specialist units.

True hermaphrodites

In true hermaphroditism and in the presence of a Y chromosome with internal genitalia and female sex of rearing, laparoscopy is indicated to inspect the internal genitalia (gonads and uterus) and to biopsy or remove gonadal tissue incompatible with the assigned sex.

THERAPY

From the outset the physician should explain to the parents that there is some doubt concerning the sex of the infant and that further investigations are needed. The parents must be told to delay registration of the child until there is certainty about the sex of rearing. If the phallus is so small that after discus-sion with an experienced pediatric surgeon surgical correction and hormonal treatment are not expected to result in a normally functioning penis, the parents should be told that the child *is* a girl.

If uncertainty exists because the phallus is of reasonable size or the degree of testosterone responsiveness is not yet known (particularly if gonads are present in the scrotal-labial folds) the decision on sex of rearing should be postponed until further investigation results are available or after a trial of testosterone therapy. This period, however, should be kept as short as possible, as it is extremely difficult for the parents to live with uncertainty about the sex of their baby.

Psychological support and counseling are essential and much attention should be directed towards this neglected aspect of care. Preferably a psychologist or social worker should be involved. The parents should be informed about the nature of the disorder and its consequences and receive formal genetic advice. Generally there is a good prognosis for living a normal life, including normal sexual activity.

Female sex of rearing

Therapy is dependent on the precise diagnosis. One of the first actions should be to normalize the external genitalia. If a female sex is assigned and the clitoris is enlarged, it has to be reduced by cliteroplasty, preserving the venous and nervous supply to the glans (**6.35, 6.36**). If there is complete or partial fusion of the labial folds, either a one-stage or two-stage operation program can be designed. Highly specialized surgeons tend to perform vaginoplasty early in the patient's life and to ensure connection to the uterus, if present (for example in congenital adrenal hyperplasia). Others may perform initial cliteroplasty together with a separation of the fused labia, and at puberty perform vaginoplasty and connection to the uterus, if required. If necessary, the vagina can be

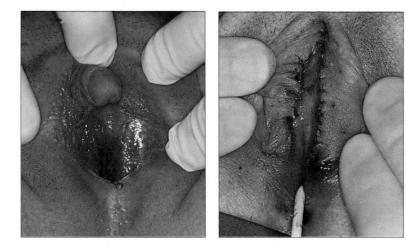

6.35, 6.36 Late presenting simple virilizing 21-hydroxylase deficiency, (height SDS + 1.8, chronological age 7.5 years, bone age 14.7 years). Pre- and post-cliteroplasty. In this case the vaginal orifice was adequate and no later surgery was required. (The stage 5 pubic hair has been shaved off.)

widened by regular use of dilators in collaboration with a gynecologist.

In all cases of congenital adrenal hyperplasia, treatment with hydrocortisone is indicated to suppress ACTH levels and to maintain normal growth rate and skeletal maturation. This treatment and its monitoring is highly specialized and should be confined to experienced centers. Some authorities recommend the use of regular multiple daily profiles of 17α-hydroxyprog-

esterone, androstenedione and plasma renin activity to monitor control (by confirming day-long suppression). Others use only regular (at least 6 monthly) measurement of bone age coupled with accurate estimations of height velocity to monitor control (a raised height velocity >50%, and rapidly advancing bone age >chronological advance, demonstrate undertreatment; a low height velocity usually indicates overtreatment or other pathology (**6.37, 6.38.**).

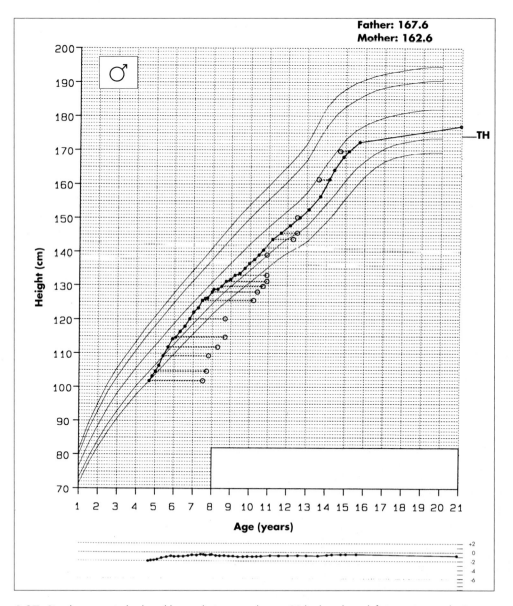

6.37 Simple congenital adrenal hyperplasia secondary to 21-hydroxylase deficiency in a male. Bone age 7.5 years at 4.8 years of age with height –2 SDS, within target range but with evidence of early virilization. With hydrocortisone replacement therapy there is an improvement in height to –1 SDS, within the target range and a gradual normalization of the bone age.

In neonates with 21-hydroxylase deficiency the hydrocortisone dosage is often close to 30 mg/m²/day. Later it can gradually be decreased to 15–25 mg/m²/day, and 12–15 mg/m²/day from 2 years onwards. Hydrocortisone should be divided as a three times a day dose, usually divided 2:1:1 or 1:1:2 to mimic the normal diurnal secretion of cortisol.

In those forms of congenital adrenal hyperplasia in which salt loss is present, either clinically or sub-clinically (i.e. detected only by elevated plasma renin activity (PRA) levels, see Chapter 8), then 9α-fluorocortisone (fludrocortisone acetate) should be added at a dose between 0.15–0.25 mg/m²/day. The dose should be adjusted by measurement of blood pressure and PRA. (Elevated PRA means that the dosage should be increased, a low PRA indicates over-treatment.) At the time of diagnosis, in hot weather and in some severely affected individuals,

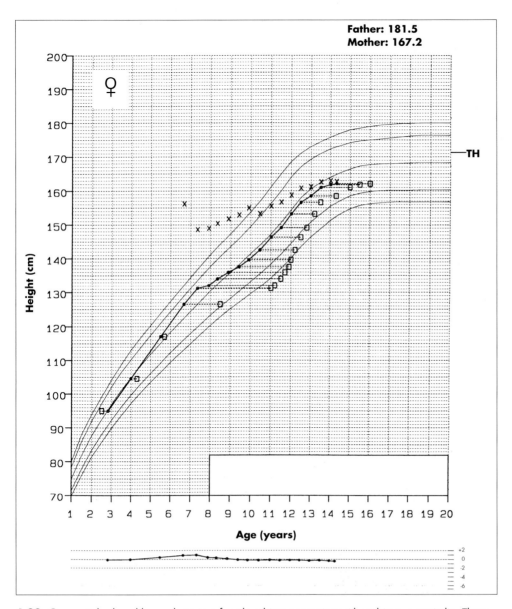

6.38 Congenital adrenal hyperplasia in a female subject presenting with ambiguous genitalia. There is evidence of under-treatment between 5.5 and 7.4 years with an advancing bone age and increased height velocity indicating non-suppression of testosterone levels. There is subsequent regaining of control with gradual improvement of height prediction but a mildly reduced final height in relation to the target range.

sodium chloride, 1 g per 10 kg body weight, may also be needed. Adequate salt and mineralocorticoid replacement is necessary to achieve satisfactory overall control.

If there is presence of even a portion of a normal ovary then secondary sex characteristics should develop at puberty (although fertility will be less certain). In cases of prolonged exposure to high androgen levels, for instance in late presenting congenital adrenal hyperplasia, a polycystic change may occur in the ovaries leading to dysmenorrhea and later hirsutism, even in the presence of adequate replacement therapy. If no ovarian tissue is present, estrogen treatment is necessary from around 10 years of age (see Chapter 5).

In the more complete forms of androgen insensitivity syndrome, the testes are removed either in early life or after puberty, as there is an increased risk for later malignancy. The presence of testes at puberty allows for some normal female sexual development without medication as testosterone is converted by aromatase to estrogen. However, the risk of malignancy before puberty, though very small, may still be considered too high to accept and gonadectomy is increasingly performed in early life. Estrogen treatment is then necessary for the development of female secondary characteristics (see Chapter 5).

Male sex of rearing

To normalize the external genitalia initially a hypospadias repair may need to be performed in one or several stages depending on the severity of the defect. Vaginal remnants and any internal female structures can also be removed. Orchidopexy, again either in one or several stages, should bring the testes to the scrotum, if possible. If the testes are internal and there is no possibility of successful orchidopexy to bring them to a position where they can be examined externally, then careful consideration should be given to gonadectomy to remove the potential risk of later undetected malignant change.

Testosterone injections (25 mg testosterone esters i.m., every 3 weeks on three occasions) can be given to increase the infant's penile size. Topical testosterone cream, 2.5% for three months, may also prove effective (but if applied by female carers they must wear gloves).

At puberty in the absence of functioning testes, testosterone replacement treatment is required. A mixture of testosterone esters given as a depot intramuscular injection is commonly used, which gives acceptable testosterone levels for about 3–4 weeks. This treatment is started at approximately 12–13 years of age and the dosage is slowly increased from

50 mg to 250 mg every 3–4 weeks. Even a relatively small, damaged testicular remnant may be able to produce sufficient testosterone to allow spontaneous virilization (**5.3**) although fertility will be unlikely.

In those cases due to forms of congenital adrenal hyperplasia, replacement therapy as outlined above should be commenced at diagnosis.

MICROPENIS

Micropenis is defined as a stretched penile length of more than 2 SD below the average for age. This equates to less than 2 cm at birth and less than 4 cm before normal puberty. The stretched penile length is measured by taking a wooden spatula and pressing it alongside the penis onto the pubic bone. A mark is then made at the level of the top of the penile glans and the length measured (**6.39**). This procedure is to ensure that the part of the penis that is buried in the subcutaneous fat is being measured. A 'hidden' penis may be misdiagnosed as micropenis unless this technique is used.

ETIOLOGY

Micropenis can be caused by hypogonadotropic hypogonadism, either isolated or in combination with other pituitary deficiencies, especially GH deficiency. It is also seen in cases of primary hypogonadism and in incomplete forms of the androgen insensitivity syndrome.

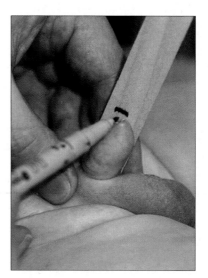

6.39
Measurement of stretched penile length.

DIAGNOSTIC WORK-UP

Initially exclude pituitary dysfunction. This can be done by measuring serum (F)T4 and TSH, as well as a 0900 serum cortisol. (Before 3 months of age there is no circadian rhythm and 3 or 4 random levels or a Synacthen test can be used as a substitute.) Low basal values are suggestive of other pituitary problems. If hypoglycemia occurs (see Chapter 8) take blood for cortisol and growth hormone. If the cortisol value is abnormally low, the diagnosis is likely to be hypopituitarism without the need for further stimulation tests. A rise in GH in response to hypoglycemia may not always occur in the neonatal period and the GH axis should thus be re-evaluated if there is evidence of later faltering of growth.

If the infant is seen between birth and 4 months of age, a basal serum testosterone measurement is useful, as in this period there is a physiological rise with a peak at 8 weeks. A normal testosterone level rules out a serious disorder of testicular androgen secretion. Also during the first 4 months (and in the pubertal age range) measurements of basal serum LH and FSH may be useful. Grossly elevated values indicate primary gonadal failure and undetectable levels indicate the need for further testing.

At any other age, or if the base-line testosterone result is low or inconclusive, a short hCG test is performed taking testosterone and DHT levels 3 days after the injection, (see Appendix A). A rise in testosterone and DHT indicates normal testicular function and 5α-reductase activity.

Outside the first 4 months basal levels of LH and FSH are also not very helpful and although a GnRH test can be performed (see Appendix A), the results often do not provide certainty about the differentiation between hypogonadotropic hypogonadism and normal function (see Chapter 5).

THERAPY

Micropenis should be treated by a series of three or four depot i.m. injections of testosterone esters or topical testosterone as described above. In infants and small children the injectable dosage is 25 mg (and larger doses can be given at puberty). If the micropenis is associated with cryptorchidism it may be more appropriate to use hCG or gonadotropins for 2-3 months to try to achieve testicular descent and penile growth from endogenous secretion of testosterone (see below). If there is poor response in terms of growth of the penis, a form of androgen insensitivity is likely and in extreme cases a lack of response

in infancy may give rise to reconsideration of the decision about sex of rearing. Late presenting cases who respond poorly have the unsatisfactory options of augmentative surgery or gender reassignment.

CRYPTORCHIDISM

ETIOLOGY

If the testes are impalpable in a phenotypic male (**6.40**) one should always first consider the possibility of an XX individual with severe female pseudo-hermaphroditism.

Simple cryptorchidism is however common. In premature babies, the testes can still descend during the first year of life. Cryptorchidism may be caused by either mechanical factors or a failure of the normal hormonal environment. It is seen with increased frequency in:
- Gonadotropin deficiency.
- Testicular dysgenesis, including chromosomal abnormalities.
- Association with other congenital malformations and syndromes.

DIAGNOSTIC WORK-UP

Medical history and physical examination
The history should concentrate on maternal health and treatment during pregnancy, mode and time of delivery and family history of genital abnormalities. In later presenting cases one should ask about the sense of smell and mental development (see Chapter 5).

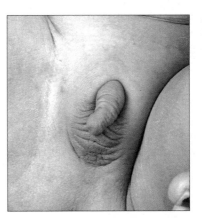

6.40 Congenital anorchia.

The physical examination should exclude other dysmorphic features or malformations and be performed both in the supine and squatting position. The maximal descent of the testes is noted and the ease of retraction after manipulation. Highly retractile testes can mimic maldescent.

Interpretation of the clues
Impalpable testes
- With no other abnormalities = simple cryptorchidism, anorchia, female pseudo-hermaphroditism.
- + micropenis with or without hypospadias = partial androgen synthesis or insensitivity syndromes.
- + anosmia and micropenis = the Kallmann syndrome.
- + mental retardation or dysmorphic features = syndromic abnormality.
- + micropenis and/or mid-line defects = gonadotropin deficiency.
- Above + neonatal hypoglycemia = multiple pituitary hormone deficiency.
- + tall stature (testes may be high in the inguinal canal and small and firm) = the Klinefelter syndrome.

THERAPY

Orchidopexy is performed if there is cryptorchidism with no possibility of descent when assessed by an experienced surgeon. The optimum time of operation is debated but is usually performed at around 2-3 years. If there is any doubt about the possibility of descent, and in cases of presumed central gonadotropin deficiency, a course of hCG can be given (500 U twice a week i.m. for 5 weeks between 1–6 years of age, and 1000 U twice a week in later childhood). If there is no satisfactory result, surgery is necessary.

MISCELLANEOUS GENITAL ABNORMALITIES

Many variations on normal anatomy exist in both sexes. They are usually spontaneous malformations although they may be associated with other syndromic abnormalities.

The male may have a shawl scrotum (**1.102**) with or without a bifid appearance. The shaft of the penis may be completely within the scrotal skin and require operative release. These abnormalities may be isolated or as part of a chromosomal abnormality (**6.41, 6.42**) or eponymous syndrome (**6.43, 6.44**). Hypospadias and epispadias are usually isolated, but severe hypospadias (**6.45**) may represent the incomplete form of androgen insensitivity syndrome. Other bizarre abnormalities, including reversed genitalia (**6.46**) and trifid scrotum (**6.47**), may also occur.

In the female there may be complete absence of the uterus and vagina (**6.48**). The hymen may be imperforate or there may be a transverse vaginal septum, both of which may present early with distension or late with hydrocolpos (**6.49**) or primary amenorrhea. (**6.50–6.52**). If vaginal abnormalities are associated with renal and / or skeletal abnormalities this forms the Rokitansky syndrome. Labial adhesions are a common finding and of no pathological significance

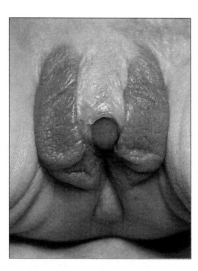

6.41 Shawl scrotum with abnormal phallus and midline cloaca, secondary to trisomy 16 with a deletion of the short arm of chromosome 5.

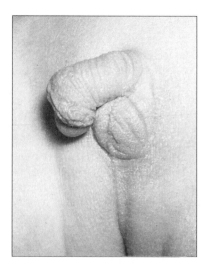

6.42 45XX + ring chromosome with hypospadias and cryptorchidism.

(**6.53**). They resolve spontaneously and surgical intervention should be discouraged. Topical treatment with estrogen cream will result in resolution but with local pigmentation as a side effect.

PRENATAL MANAGEMENT OF 21-HYDROXYLASE DEFICIENCY

As 21-hydroxylase deficiency is an autosomal recessive disease the risk for subsequent siblings of an affected proband is 25%. The most serious consequence of the disorder is the genital ambiguity in females. Therefore it is most important to prevent masculinization of the external genitalia in affected female fetuses. The following strategy has been developed in specialist centers.

Identifying the HLA genotype of the index case and parents along with the restriction fragment length polymorphisms (RFLP) of the 21-hydroxylase gene will allow for later identification of affected fetuses in informative kindreds. The mother is instructed to start dexamethasone therapy at a dose of 20 μg per kg body weight per day when she is sure she is pregnant. A chorionic biopsy is performed at 9–10 weeks gestation or amniocentesis at 15–18 weeks which allows the fetus to be sexed and the HLA type and genotype assessed. If the fetus is female *and* affected dexamethasone is continued throughout pregnancy, otherwise treatment is discontinued. After birth the infant is carefully reassessed and treatment with hydrocortisone and 9α-fluorocortisone is commenced if the diagnosis is confirmed.

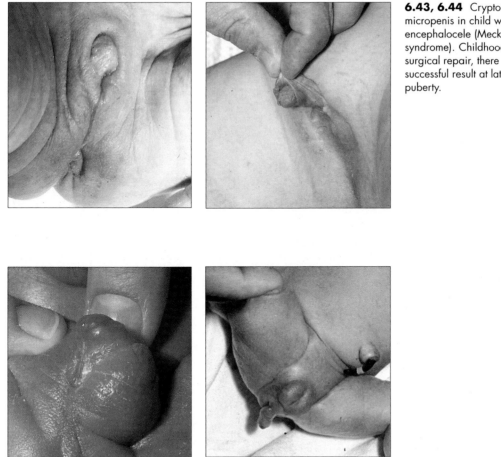

6.43, 6.44 Cryptorchidism and micropenis in child with posterior encephalocele (Meckel–Gruber syndrome). Childhood outcome of surgical repair, there was a fairly successful result at later induced puberty.

6.45 Severe hypospadias and micropenis, 46XY.

6.46 Reversed male genitalia.

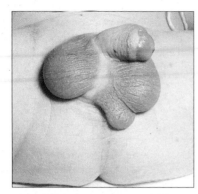

6.47 Trifid scrotum, cause unknown.

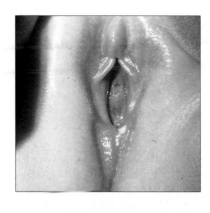

6.48 Vaginal atresia, uterus also absent.

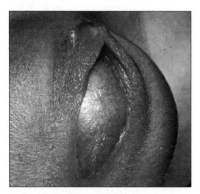

6.49 Hydrocolpos secondary to transverse vaginal septum.

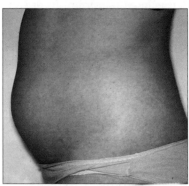

6.50 Imperforate hymen presenting as primary amenorrhea with abdominal distension.

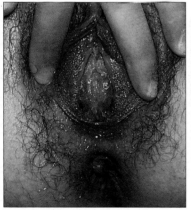

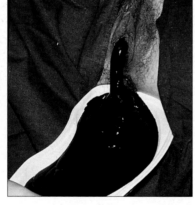

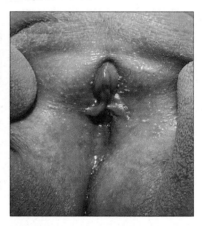

6.51, 6.52 Same case at operation showing bluish discoloration of imperforate hymen and resulting discharge of old blood following surgical incision.

6.53 Labial adhesions. Spontaneous resolution will always occur.

7.

Goiter

ASSESSMENT OF THYROID SIZE AND FUNCTION

The thyroid can be best palpated whilst standing behind the sitting patient or with the patient lying with the head falling backwards slightly over the edge of the couch. For accurate documentation of size one practical method is to draw a line on the skin around the contours of the thyroid gland and to copy this onto a sheet of thin plastic. This plastic can be stored in the case records so that the size can be assessed longitudinally.

Thyromegaly (**7.1**) can occur as a result of stimulation, infiltration, or inflammation and can be diffuse or nodular (localized) (**7.2**).

ETIOLOGY

- **Endemic iodine deficiency** is the main cause of goiter, either euthyroid or with hypothyroidism, in areas of the world with poor natural sources of iodine and in the absence of a salt supplementation program.
- **Autoimmune thyroiditis (Hashimoto disease)** is the commonest cause of goiter in non-iodine deficient areas. The pathogenesis of this disorder is uncertain, but a deficiency in antigen-specific sup-

pressor T lymphocytes may be present. Anti-thyroid antibodies are usually present in high titers. It can be associated with other autoimmune disorders and antibodies against adrenal cortex, parathyroid, gastric parietal cells, etc (polyglandular syndrome type 1, 2 or 2) (**7.3**, **1.66**, **3.17**, **3.33**). Patients with euthyroid Hashimoto disease should be followed for a few years to see if they develop hypo- or hyperthyroidism (see below).

- **Idiopathic simple goiter or adolescent goiter** (**7.4**, **7.5**), the enlargement of the gland at the time of puberty to form a visible goiter, is not uncommon in euthyroid individuals, often with a positive family

7.1 Goiter.

Causes of thyromegaly

Diffuse Thyromegaly	Nodular Thyromegaly
Autoimmune thyroiditis (Hashimoto disease)	Autoimmune thyroiditis
Thyrotoxicosis (Graves disease)	Simple thyroid cyst
Toxic thyroiditis (Hashitoxicosis)	Thyroid tumors:-
Idiopathic (simple) thyromegaly	Adenoma (hyper-functioning [hot], or non-functioning [cold])
Iodine deficiency in endemic areas	Carcinoma (MTC or papillary)
Goitrogen ingestion	Other tumors
Antithyroid drugs	Non-thyroidal masses
Familial dyshormonogenesis	Lymphadenopathy
Acute and subacute thyroiditis	Branchial cleft cyst
TSH secreting pituitary adenoma (very rare)	Thyroglossal duct cyst
Pituitary resistance to thyroid hormone (PRTH) (very rare)	

7.2 Causes of thyromegaly.

history of goiter. Regression is usual but nodular changes may occur three or four decades later.

- **Thyrotoxicosis.**
- **Acute bacterial thyroiditis** with fever and tenderness.
- **Sub-acute thyroiditis** with lymphocytic infiltration, tenderness and often evidence of intercurrent upper respiratory tract infection.
- **Ingestion of goitrogens** either as anti-thyroid drugs or as naturally occurring compounds in the diet, such as large amounts of soya and cabbage.
- **Unidentified agents** in specific geographical areas can induce goiter.
- **Dyshormonogenesis** which usually presents as goitrous neonatal hypothyroidism (see below) but may occasionally present with goiter in later life.

Hypo- and hyperthyroidism will now be discussed as the most important clinical causes of goiter; congenital hypothyroidism with or without goiter is discussed in Chapter 8.

The polyglandular syndromes

Type	Features
Type 1	Two or more of: Candidiasis, hypoparathyroidism, Addisonism.
Type 2	Addisonism plus: Type 1 diabetes mellitus. And/or Thyroid antibodies.
Type 3a	Thyroid antibodies plus Type 1 diabetes mellitus.
Type 3b	Thyroid antibodies plus pernicious anemia.
Type 3c	Thyroid antibodies plus vitiligo and alopecia plus other autoimmune disease.

Vitiligo can be a component of any of the syndromes.

7.3 The polyglandular syndromes.

JUVENILE HYPOTHYROIDISM

This occurs most commonly in Hashimoto disease. It is also strongly associated with several syndromes with abnormal karyotype such as the Ullrich–Turner, Klinefelter and Down syndrome (where there is also an increased incidence of thyroid dysgenesis, see Chapter 8); with non-chromosomal disorders, for instance the Noonan syndrome and also metabolic disorders such as cystinosis.

History and examination

The exploration of the presenting history of suspected hypothyroidism should include:

- Family history of over- or underactive thyroid glands, any other familial autoimmune disease.
- A history of recent growth failure and any tendency to weight gain.
- Any tiredness or weakness?
- Any change in activity levels, school performance or mental state?
- Constipation?
- Any hair loss or changes in the skin?
- Heat preference and intolerance of cold?
- Deepening of the voice?
- In females post menarche, any menstrual irregularity or long, heavy periods?

On examination search for:

- Height reduced in relation to weight centile.
- Back relatively longer than the legs.
- If old records exist, low height velocity.
- Goiter (not always present).
- Delayed or arrested puberty *or* advanced sexual maturation. (In boys manifested by enlarging testicles and penis with little hair growth and in females by sexual precocity and cystic ovarian changes.)
- Myxedema (rare in childhood).
- Dry skin, vitiligo (**7.6**).
- Deep voice.

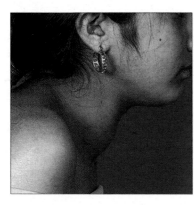
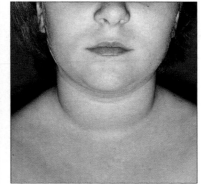

7.4, 7.5 Two cases of simple pubertal goiter.

- Hair loss, often in the temporal area (**7.7**, **7.8**).
- Proximal weakness and delayed relaxation of the tendon reflexes.

Rarely the pituitary may enlarge because of hypertrophy of the thyrotrophin producing cells, and produce visual field loss from optic chiasm compression (**7.9**).

DIAGNOSTIC WORK-UP

For the detection of hypothyroidism, serum free T_4 (FT_4) and TSH measurements are most valuable. (If no FT_4 assay is available, total T_4 can be used, but one should bear in mind that the total T_4 level is largely determined by the thyroxine binding globulin (TBG) concentration. The TBG level can be assayed and is low in congenital deficiency without any clinical consequences. Thus, a low total T_4 does not necessarily indicate hypothyroidism, see Chapter 8.) The combination of a low $(F)T_4$ with an elevated TSH concentration is proof of primary hypothyroidism. Antithyroid antibodies indicate an autoimmune process in the thyroid, and are usually present in Hashimoto thyroiditis as may be antibodies to other glands in the polyendocrinopathy syndromes.

The bone age is often markedly delayed and the epiphyses are wider than normal, or eroded. In the presence of early sexual maturation the LH/ FSH ratio may be less than 1, which is abnormal (see Chapter 4).

Although with modern TSH assays this is rarely required, a TRH-test can sometimes be helpful (see Appendix A). If compensated hypothyroidism is suspected with euthyroidism at the expense of mildly elevated TSH levels there will be an exuberant rise of TSH. The test can also be used to differentiate the non-goitrous or artefactual causes of hypothyroidism. An extremely low TSH level during the whole test indicates a pituitary (secondary) deficiency. A pattern in which TSH continues to rise after 20 minutes is indicative of a hypothalamic (tertiary) defect. A normal TRH test is seen in TBG deficiency. It should be noted that secondary/tertiary hypothyroidism can show few symptoms or signs and that serum $(F)T_4$ is usually not far below the normal range. Urinary iodine excretion can be measured to document iodine deficiency.

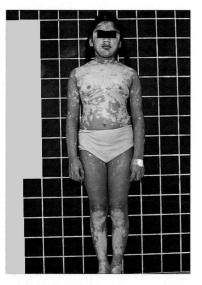

7.6 Vitiligo.

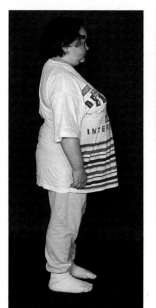

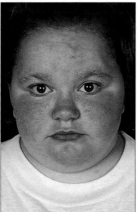

7.7, 7.8 Gross obesity and temporal hair loss in hypothyroidism. There was a weight loss of 15 kilos in the first 2 months of therapy.

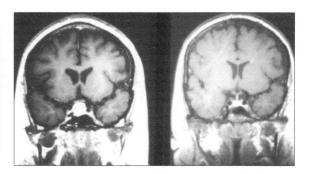

7.9 Pituitary enlargement producing compression of the optic chiasm in prolonged hypothyroidism, before and after thyroxine therapy.

THERAPY

Treatment consists of L-thyroxine in sufficient dosage to normalize serum TSH levels (which will keep the serum $(F)T_4$ in the upper normal range, or even somewhat higher). The child is checked, initially, at frequent intervals (1–3 months) and then yearly when a correct dose is determined. The dosage should be individually titrated but is usually in the order of 2–3 µg/kg/day depending on age (or around 100 µg/m²). After the onset of therapy, weight often reduces markedly (**7.10, 7.11**). Catch-up growth in height is usually seen, but final height is often not as tall as may be expected from the very delayed bone age.

THYROTOXICOSIS

This condition is almost always caused by Graves disease and the presence of thyroid stimulating antibodies. There is a strong association with infiltration of the orbit by mucopolysaccharide material that produces the characteristic eye signs. Eye disease is usually less pronounced in children than in adults and the infiltrative dermopathy seen in adults is very rare indeed in children. Thyrotoxicosis is very much more common in females and is strongly familial.

In the rare syndrome of pituitary resistance to thyroid hormones (PRTH), there is hyperthyroidism because of a lack of feedback inhibition of the pituitary. 'Hot' TSH secreting pituitary adenomas have been described but are exceedingly rare in childhood.

HISTORY AND EXAMINATION

The exploration of the presenting history of suspected hyperthyroidism should include:
- Family history of over- or underactive thyroid glands; any other familial autoimmune disease.
- A history of recent growth acceleration and any tendency to lose weight, *often in the presence of increased appetite.*
- Any tiredness or weakness?
- Any increase in activity levels or change in mental state? i.e. decreased ability to concentrate on mental tasks.
- Anxiety (and sometimes frank psychosis).
- Poor school performance.
- Fidgety foot and hand movements, generally increased activity.
- Frequent stools?
- Palpitations?
- Any diplopia, eye pain or redness?
- Cold preference and intolerance of heat?
- In females post menarche, any menstrual irregularity, scanty periods or amenorrhea?
- Any thinning of the hair?

On examination search for:
- Weight reduced in relation to height centile.
- If old records exist, increased height velocity (**3.29**).
- Goiter (**7.12**).
- Chemosis, exophthalmos, lid lag, ophthalmoplegia (**7.13, 7.14**).
- Tachycardia.

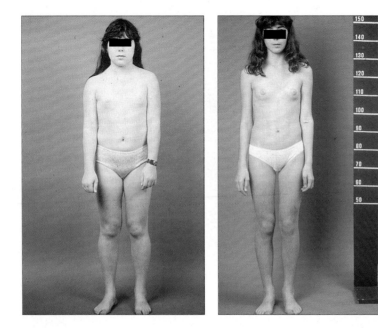

7.10, 7.11 Hypothyroidism before and 18 months after starting treatment. There has been weight loss, progression of puberty and improvement of the lank, greasy hair.

- Increased systolic and decreased diastolic blood pressure, leading to a wide pulse pressure.
- Sweatiness.
- Anxiety or abnormal behavior.
- Tremor. This is best appreciated as a buzz transmitted from the outstretched, spread fingers of the patient to the palm of the examiner's hand. It is of high frequency and may not be visible to the eye.
- Proximal weakness and brisk tendon reflexes.
- Thinning of the hair.

DIAGNOSTIC WORK-UP

Thyroid stimulating immunoglobulins (TSI), also called thyrotrophin receptor antibodies, are almost always present, but require specialized laboratories for their measurement. In clinical practice these assays are rarely necessary as the signs and symptoms are so typical. The diagnosis is confirmed by high (F)T_4 in the presence of suppressed TSH levels. New, ultra-sensitive TSH assays can distinguish a low TSH level from one in the normal range.

If used, total T_4 levels again can cause confusion in rare congenital situations of TBG excess or, more commonly, secondary to pregnancy or various drug therapies such as the contraceptive pill, where T_4 levels will appear high whilst FT_4 levels would be normal (see Chapter 8).

In rare cases of doubt, a TRH test can be done, which will show a suppressed TSH response in the earliest stages of the disease (see Appendix A).

Serum total or FT_3 can occasionally be valuable in the rare diagnosis of 'T_3 toxicosis' where FT_3 levels are raised inappropriately for the levels of FT_4 detected on standard assays.

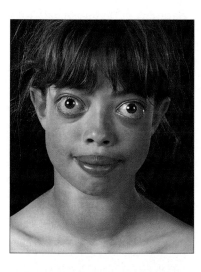

7.12 Goiter in Graves disease.

THERAPY

There are four forms of therapy. All have their advantages and disadvantages and require the supervision of an experienced endocrinologist, especially in the early stages of treatment.

1. Symptomatic relief

In addition to therapies directed against the thyroid itself, it may be necessary in the early stages of treatment, before lowered FT_4 levels are achieved, to administer a β-blocker, usually propanolol at a three times a day dose of 1–2 mg/kg, to alleviate the symptoms of hyperthyroidism. This strategy cannot be used in the presence of a history of asthma.

2. Antithyroid drugs

Propylthiouracil (PTU), methimazole, and carbimazole may be used. PTU may have the theoretical advantage of blocking peripheral conversion of T_4 to T_3 and that

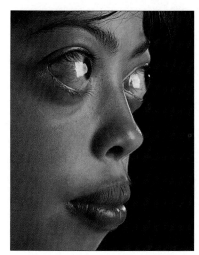
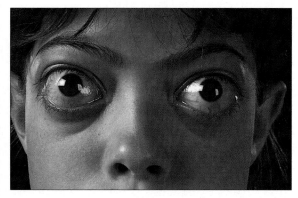

7.13, 7.14 Exophthalmos and chemosis in Graves disease.

it may reduce the titers of thyrotrophin receptor anti-bodies. It is also less likely to exacerbate hair loss if this is a presenting feature of the condition. It is given in a dosage of 5–10 mg/kg/day in 3 divided doses. The equivalent dosages for methimazole and carbimazole are approximately one tenth of the PTU dosage.

There is some evidence that the chances of later relapse are reduced if the antithyroid drugs are given at a dose sufficient to suppress FT_4 and in combination with L-thyroxine at a replacement dose. This 'blocking' regime also has the advantage that it is not necessary constantly to increase and decrease drug dosage to try to titrate anti-thyroid therapy to maintain euthyroid FT_4 levels.

Therapy is usually continued for between 6 months to 2 years, after which remission is achieved in about 50% of cases. The dosage can then be slowly tapered. If relapse occurs, antithyroid therapy may be resumed or the patient may be offered the choice of surgical or radio-iodine therapy (see below). The major disadvantages of drug therapy are its long duration, compliance with what may be a three times a day dose regime, and the risk of toxic side effects (**7.15**). These require the estimation of full blood count in the first 4 weeks of therapy when myelotoxicity is most likely to occur. If any serious side effects are suspected therapy must be stopped immediately.

3. Subtotal thyroidectomy

This can be occasionally a first-line therapy but is more commonly used in cases of relapse after initial drug treatment. The surgeon must have experience of this procedure in children. Permanent hypoparathyroidism and damage to the recurrent laryngeal nerve are possible hazards of surgical intervention.

4. Iodine[131] treatment

This has the advantage that it is effective in around 85% of patients and once administered requires merely surveillance for the development of later hypothyroidism (20% within one year increasing to around 60% after a decade). There are few short-term risks and 40 years of experience in some centers indicates that there is little risk of later malignant change. It should, however, be considered only in experienced centers.

Treatment of the eye disease is rarely required in childhood. Occasionally, intra-ocular steroid injections or surgical decompression may be necessary to preserve vision.

In some cases of Graves disease there are detectable levels of anti-thyroid antibodies of the same kind as found in Hashimoto thyroiditis. In these cases spontaneous hypothyroidism may ensue after initial toxicosis, so-called 'Hashitoxicosis'.

NEONATAL THYROTOXICOSIS

If mothers with Graves disease become pregnant the circulating thyrotrophin receptor antibodies can cross the placenta in the last trimester and cause fetal thyrotoxicosis. This is *not* dependent on the current thyroid status of the mother (the antibodies persist after spontaneous or therapeutically induced hypothyroidism) and so obstetric staff should be alert to the possibility in any mother with a history suggestive of thyrotoxicosis.

The incidence is approximately 1 in 25×10^3 pregnancies. During pregnancy, fetal size and heart rate have to be closely monitored. In case of fetal tachycardia, low dose PTU (25–50 mg) can be given to the mother to treat the fetus *in utero*. If the mother is being treated with antithyroid drugs, these can also cross the placenta and cause fetal hypothyroidism and goiter (**7.16**).

Whether or not fetal thyrotoxicosis has been detected and treated *in utero*, after birth the infant may develop the symptoms of thyrotoxicosis with tachycardia, hyperkinesis, restlessness, diarrhea, poor weight gain, premature craniostenosis and advanced bone age (**7.17**). The diagnosis is confirmed by high $(F)T_4$ and suppressed TSH levels. As the maternally administered antithyroid drugs will be metabolized by the 5th day, but the TSI will persist for 3–5 months, the neonate requires frequent reassessment in the first ten days of life.

Therapy is with PTU (5–10 mg/kg) and propanolol (2 mg/kg) to achieve symptomatic control or alternatively saturated potassium iodide (Lugol's solution) at one drop every 8 hours.

Side effects of antithyroid drugs

Rashes (common, exchange drugs or, if no substitution possible, treat with anti-histamines and continue therapy)

Nausea

Headache

Pruritus

Arthralgia

Alopecia (less with PTU)

Jaundice

Lupus (with PTU)

Agranulocytosis: patient told to report *any* symptoms of infection, especially sore throat, as soon as they occur. A white cell count should be immediately checked and therapy discontinued if there is *any* clinical or laboratory suggestion of neutropenia.

7.15 Side effects of antithyroid drugs propylthiouracil (PTU), carbimazole and methimazole.

AUTONOMOUS THYROID NODULE

Thyroid nodules in childhood are rare (**7.18**). They are often not associated with hormone excess but may occasionally produce thyrotoxicosis and require surgical removal. It is wise to consider needle biopsy in all cases to exclude papillary carcinoma of the thyroid.

THYROID CARCINOMA

Papillary carcinoma usually presents as an asymmetric thyroid mass in teenage life. There may be anti-thyroid antibodies present. The carcinoma is often metastatic at presentation but the prognosis is excellent in childhood. Treatment involves thyroidectomy followed by I^{131} treatment and then complete suppression of TSH levels by L-Thyroxine. The cells are well differentiated and produce thyroglobulin which can be used as a marker of the disease process. The outlook with adequate treatment and monitoring is excellent.

Medullary cell carcinoma is almost always a component of MEA 2 or 2b. Diagnosis of this condition on clinical presentation of other components of the syndrome (**7.19**) should prompt immediate removal of the thyroid gland as the risk of malignant change is so great. It is now possible to screen relatives of affected individuals by DNA analysis for abnormalities of the *ret* oncogene on chromosome 10q, in informative families, to allow pre-symptomatic thyroid resection.

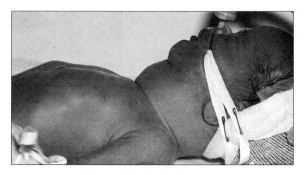

7.16 Neonatal goitre secondary to maternal PTU treatment for thyrotoxicosis. The goiter has compressed the trachea, requiring endotracheal intubation to maintain the airway.

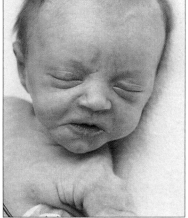

7.17 Neonatal thyrotoxicosis.

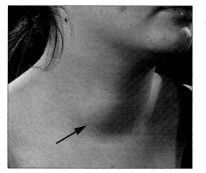

7.18 'Cold' thyroid nodule.

The multiple endocrine adenomatosis (MEA) syndromes

Syndrome	Components
MEA 1	Parathyroid, pituitary & pancreatic adenomas (prolactinomas).
MEA 2a	Medullary cell carcinoma of the thyroid, pheochromocytoma, parathyroid adenomas.
MEA 2b	Medullary cell carcinoma of the thyroid, pheochromocytoma, mucosal neuromas, intestinal neuronal dysplasia, marfanoid habitus.

Familial medullary cell carcinoma of the thyroid.

7.19 The multiple endocrine adenomatosis (MEA) or multiple endocrine neoplasia (MEN) syndromes.

8.

Abnormal Laboratory Values

CONGENITAL HYPOTHYROIDISM

The majority of infants with congenital hypothyroidism present as a result of routine neonatal screening and hence will be discussed in this chapter.

PHYSIOLOGY

During fetal life the thyroid starts to produce thyroid hormone from 20 weeks onwards, stimulated by pituitary TSH secretion. Thyroxine (T_4) is first metabolized primarily to inactive reverse triiodothyronine (rT_3) by the placenta and only after 30 weeks does the active T_3 level start to rise. It was thought for many years that maternal T_4 does not cross the placenta but recently there is evidence that some T_4 can pass to the fetal circulation. The majority of release of thyroid hormones from the thyroid gland is in the form of T_4 which is deiodinated to T_3 in the peripheral tissues or deactivated by the formation of rT_3 and then further deiodination. Most of the activity of the hormones is mediated by the action of T_3 on intranuclear receptors. Normal levels of thyroid hormones in infancy and childhood are given in Appendix B.

Congenital hypothyroidism can be divided into primary, secondary and tertiary forms. Primary hypothyroidism is caused either by embryonic defects (agenesis, dysgenesis, ectopia) and accounts for 95% of cases, or by dyshormonogenesis. This latter category comprises several enzyme deficiencies which are usually transmitted as an autosomal recessive trait. Secondary or tertiary hypothyroidism is usually associated with other pituitary hormone deficiencies and accounts for only 1–2% of cases.

The Down syndrome is associated with an increased incidence of thyroid agenesis.

CLINICAL FINDINGS

In most developed nations all neonates are screened for hypothyroidism. The cost–benefit ratio is high, as the incidence is around 1 in 4×10^3 and early detection and treatment prevents later cretinism. Many affected children are asymptomatic in the first months of life. Thyrotrophin (TSH) screening is the simplest and least expensive strategy with a low number of false-positive results. With such screening secondary and tertiary hypothyroidism are not detected, but these account for only a small proportion of cases and are often detected on the basis of other clinical features of pituitary dysfunction (such as prolonged jaundice, micropenis, hypoglycemia).

Because of screening the majority of infants are asymptomatic at diagnosis. The signs which may be evident soon after birth and the signs which can further develop if the diagnosis is not made early are shown in **8.1**. These physical features will regress on treatment (**8.2–8.5**), but the later the therapy is commenced the worse is the outlook for normal mental development. Full-blown cretinism with severe mental retardation, dwarfing and the characteristic facial features (**8.6**) is now rarely seen in the developed world.

Neonatal goiter (**8.7, 7.12**) will be present in dyshormonogenesis but not in thyroid dysplasia or secondary and tertiary hypothyroidism.

Signs and symptoms in congenital hypothyroidism

Early symptoms (all or none of these may be present in the first month of life)	Late symptoms (1 month plus)
Umbilical hernia	Persists
Pallor and hypothermia	Persists
Enlarged tongue	Increases to 100%
Hypotonia	Worsens
Prolonged jaundice	Decreases
Rough, dry skin	Persists
Open posterior fontanelle	Closes
Relative constipation	Persists
Mild post-maturity Birth weight >3.5 kg	
	Facial puffiness
	Hoarse cry
	Growth retardation
	Poor development
	Myxedema

8.1 Signs and symptoms in congenital hypothyroidism.

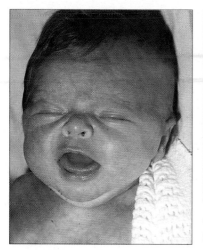

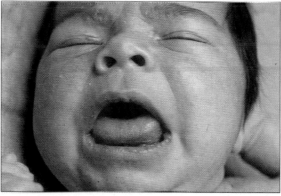

8.2, 8.3 Two cases of congenital hypothyroidism at presentation (1 month).

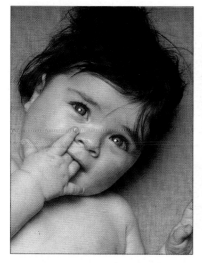

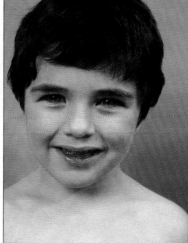

8.4, 8.5 The same case of congenital hypothyroidism as shown in **8.3** after 5 months of therapy and at 2 years of age.

8.6 Cretinism.

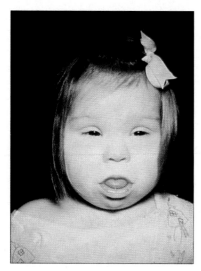

8.7 Neonatal goiter.

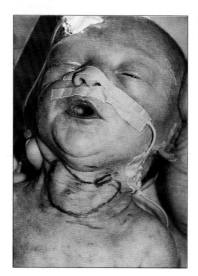

Occasionally, dyshormonogenesis can present in later childhood, and especially in the Pendred syndrome (see below) where the onset of hypothyroidism can be very variable.

DIAGNOSTIC WORK-UP

From an X-ray of the knee and foot the skeletal age can be assessed, which is usually delayed. A radio-iodine scan or technetium scan (which delivers a lower radiation dose) can visualize the thyroid, so that agenesis or ectopia can be demonstrated. This is not necessary in most straightforward cases of congenital hypothyroidism.

Radiography and ultrasonography of the thyroid by an experienced radiologist can assist in the detection of the thyroid gland and in assessing its size (**8.8**, **8.9**).

If dyshormonogenesis is suspected the radio-iodine scan (but not technetium) will provide information about causality. If there is failure of uptake of iodine into salivary or thyroid tissue then there is a defect in the concentration of iodine. This rare disorder carries a poor prognosis even with therapy. If organification is defective because of an enzyme deficiency, a perchlorate discharge test may be performed (**8.10**). The perchlorate ion will compete with iodide for trapping by the thyroid follicular cell plasma membrane and discharge of iodine will occur that can be monitored by release of radiation from the gland. If discharge occurs then the child and family should be screened for asymptomatic goiter or hypothyroidism and high tone deafness, the Pendred syndrome, which can have very variable expression in different members of a kindred. If uptake occurs and there is no discharge, then one of the other enzyme defects causing failure of de-iodination, storage or transport of thyroid hormones is present. In specialized laboratories serum thyroglobulin levels can be measured. There is no practical reason to differentiate between these conditions.

THERAPY

The first task of the physician is to treat the hypothyroid infant as soon as possible. Treatment should be started immediately. A diagnosis made on neonatal

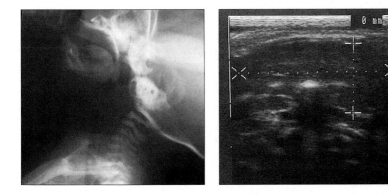

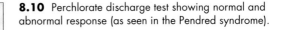

8.8, 8.9 Lateral neck radiograph showing neonatal goiter enveloping trachea. Ultrasound scan of same case, trachea in center of film, goiter measuring 35 mm by at least 16 mm.

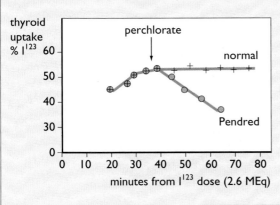

8.10 Perchlorate discharge test showing normal and abnormal response (as seen in the Pendred syndrome).

screening should be confirmed by low $(F)T_4$ and elevated TSH levels. Whilst awaiting these results, L-thyroxine is started in a dosage of 10–15 µg/kg body weight and then tapered to 7–5 µg/kg to maintain the $(F)T_4$ at the higher end of the age specific normal range and maintain a normal TSH. Over-treatment can lead to craniostenosis. In some cases the TSH levels may remain high for many months, despite adequate treatment, because of acquired hypothalamic feedback insensitivity. In rare cases of mistaken screening-based diagnosis, therapy can be discontinued with no ill effect. Therapy is continued life-long, although there is an argument for reinvestigating the occasional case where early control is achieved and when no high levels of TSH are detected during the first 2 years of follow-up (for instance because of non-compliance or inadequate dosage with growth). In this situation brief (2 week) discontinuation of therapy and the demonstration of a rising TSH will demonstrate that the hypothyroidism persists. If this TSH rise does not occur, then, occasionally, the early defect will prove to have been transient and due to maternal goitrogens or placental transfer of TSH blocking antibodies and treatment can be discontinued. If the TSH rises to a level at the upper end of the normal range with a FT_4 at the lower end of the range (evidence of compensated hypothyroidism), a technetium scan may demonstrate a small mid-line or lingual gland (**8.11**). L-thyroxine should then be recommened to remove the theoretical risk of later malignant change from chronic TSH hyperstimulation.

HYPO- AND HYPERNATREMIA

WATER REGULATION

Anatomical and physiological considerations
The osmoregulatory system is controlled by the hypothalamic neurohypophyseal axis, which includes osmoreceptors (near the supraoptic nuclei) and the neurones for the synthesis, storage and secretion of arginine vasopressin (AVP) (mainly in supraoptic nuclei, some in paraventricular nuclei). It also includes osmoreceptors of thirst, which control drinking behavior. The second component involves the kidney, where the renal collecting duct is sensitive to the action of AVP.

Arginine vasopressin secretion is controlled by changes in water balance particularly through changes in plasma osmolality, to which the osmoreceptor is extremely sensitive. The 'osmotic threshold' for the release of AVP is 280 mOsm/kg H_2O. Between 280 and 295 mOsm/kg the AVP level rises steeply.

Beyond 295 mOsm/kg AVP cannot rise further and thirst is perceived, leading to increased water intake.

The baroregulatory system is the secondary mechanism for controlling AVP secretion. The baroreceptor system (carotid sinus, aortic arch, left atrium), is much less sensitive than the osmoreceptor, since a change in blood volume of 5–10% is necessary before AVP is released. Once this threshold is exceeded, release of AVP may reach levels ten times higher than those reached after osmotic stimulation.

Hypernatremia due to diabetes insipidus (DI)
Definition and etiology
Diabetes insipidus describes different disorders of water regulation due to vasopressin deficiency or lack of action and manifested by polyuria and polydipsia with varying degrees of plasma hypertonicity. Clinical features include:
- Constipation.
- Vomiting.
- Fever.
- Loss of weight or failure to thrive.
- Dehydration.

When caused by insufficient AVP secretion this state is called central diabetes insipidus. A lack of peripheral response to AVP results in nephrogenic diabetes insipidus.

Central DI is rare in childhood and most commonly due to intracranial tumors, or as a result of neurosurgery for these tumors. Craniopharyngioma may rarely present with polyuria and polydipsia, but this is common post-operatively. Other tumors such as Langerhans' cell histiocytosis (**8.12**) and germinoma (see **2.77**) along with non-neoplastic infiltration (such as sarcoid) are also causes of DI. Mid-line anatomical defects, such as septo-optic dysplasia (see **1.109**, **1.110**) cause DI in around 30% of cases. Posterior pituitary damage can occur post-traumatically with

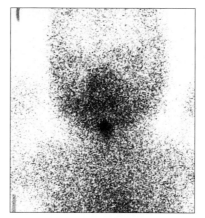

8.11 Technetium scan showing small mid-line gland in child presenting with raised TSH on screening and evidence of compensated hypothyroidism at 2 years of age.

disruption of the vulnerable pituitary stalk. The neurosecretory granules of AVP show up brightly on MRI imaging and, following stalk transection, the lesion can be demonstrated by a 'hold-up' of this material in the proximal part of the stalk (**2.80**). Idiopathic, auto-immune and familial cases also occur.

Nephrogenic DI can be inherited as an X-linked abnormality or be secondary to renal damage from metabolic disease (cystinosis, hypophosphatemia), sickle cell disease, drug therapy and chronic renal failure from any cause.

Primary polydipsia is due to a specific disorder of thirst regulation or psychogenic causes and will not result in hypernatremia.

Diagnostic work-up

The best way to differentiate the forms of diabetes insipidus (which can occur in varying degrees of severity) is a dehydration test with measurements of plasma osmolality, urine osmolality and plasma AVP (see Appendix A). If there is no AVP assay available, an acceptable alternative is a dehydration test with measurements of plasma and urine osmolality, followed by a short desmopressin (DDAVP) test.

If, after dehydration, a high plasma osmolality is found (>295 mOsm/l) with a low urine osmolality (<400 mOsm/l), there is complete central DI. Following desmopressin administration the urine osmolality increases steeply. In cases of nephrogenic DI there is only a partial rise of urine osmolality after dehydration (<800 mOsm/l) and a subnormal response to DDAVP.

Patients with primary polydipsia usually show an increase in urine osmolality during the dehydration test that is close to normal values, and administration of desmopressin causes an increase in urine osmolality of less than 10%. In some cases the test result can be abnormal after a prolonged polyuric state (due to a 'wash-out' effect in the renal medulla) and should be repeated after several days of DDAVP treatment.

Treatment

Central DI is treated with DDAVP intranasally or orally. The intranasal solution contains 0.1 mg in 1 ml. The usual daily dosage is 0.05–0.3 ml (5–30 µg) given in 2 or 3 doses. Given orally, the dosage is 10–20 times higher and tablets of 0.1 or 0.2 mg are used. The dosage should be adjusted according to response and should permit normal drinking behavior and sleep. Overdosage or continued habit polydipsia during treatment will lead to severe water intoxication and hyponatremia.

Nephrogenic DI is treated by a low solute diet, restricted protein and salt intake, and water at frequent intervals. In severe cases chlorothiazide (100 mg/m² body surface per day) can be given in three divided doses.

Hyponatremia due to inappropriate secretion of ADH

The syndrome of inappropriate secretion of ADH (SIADH) can be caused by many systemic illnesses, burns, drugs or trauma to the central nervous system. It is characterized by hyponatremia and water retention in the presence of non-dilute urine.

Treatment relies on removing the cause, if possible, combined with fluid restriction. If severe, then phenytoin (in young children) or demeclocycline (in older children) can be used, which antagonize the actions of ADH. In life-threatening situations hypertonic saline and even combinations of frusemide and fludrocortisone may be used to reverse the hyponatremia.

SALT REGULATION

Physiological considerations and laboratory tests

The renin-angiotensin-aldosterone system (RAAS) is the most important mediator in the endocrine regulation of sodium and water balance. Another component is atrial natriuretic factor which physiologically inhibits aldosteronogenesis.

The determination of plasma renin activity (PRA) is thus an important investigation in hypo- or hypernatremic states. Levels are strongly dependent on age, with the highest values in the first year of life, and also vary due to time of day, posture and sodium intake.

Aldosterone can be measured in plasma and in a 24-hour urine collection. Plasma levels are also highest in the first year of life. Diagnostic accuracy can

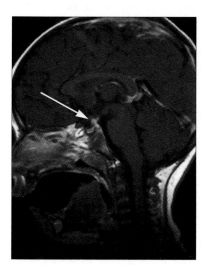

8.12 Infiltration of the pituitary stalk in Langerhans' cell histiocytosis presenting with central diabetes insipidus.

be enhanced by relating aldosterone excretion in the urine to sodium excretion.

Hyponatremia secondary to salt losing syndromes

Loss of salt occurs in gastrointestinal, renal and adrenal disorders. Gastrointestinal diseases may be easy to diagnose whereas the differential diagnosis of renal and adrenal diseases can be difficult. Clinical symptoms of salt loss comprise:

- Wasting.
- Dehydration.
- Intermittent fever.
- Salt craving.
- Shock.

Renal disease

Many chronic renal disorders can lead to salt losing states. The clinical symptoms of renal salt losing syndromes may be accompanied by the biochemical changes of proteinuria, aminoaciduria, and glycosuria. Hypokalemia due to renal loss of potassium is frequent. In infants salt loss can occur in cases of urethral obstruction with or without secondary infection and the clinical and laboratory presentation can be very similar to that of congenital adrenal hyperplasia. Sonography of the kidney and bladder is thus an important investigation in infancy accompanied by PRA and aldosterone measurements in uncertain cases.

Adrenal disorders

These comprise various defects in the synthesis of mineralocorticoid and glucocorticoid hormones (see also Chapter 6 for a discussion of congenital adrenal hyperplasia causing intersex).

In functional terms the adrenal consists of two parts: the cortex, producing steroid hormones, and the medulla, secreting catecholamines. Although interactions between both parts appear to exist, the physiologic functions can be considered as separate. In fetal life the adrenal cortex plays an important role in producing hormones which appear to be vital for placental function. After birth the adrenal cortex diminishes quickly in relative size with atrophy of the hyperplastic fetal cortex. The remaining definitive cortex consists of three layers: the outer zona glomerulosa, the zona fasciculata and the zona reticularis. There are five groups of hormones produced in the adrenal cortex: corticosteroids, mineralocorticoids, androgens, estrogens, and progestagens (**6.4**). The three groups of hormones are regulated differently. Glucocorticoid secretion is stimulated by ACTH from the pituitary in a classical negative feedback pattern. Mineralocorticoid secretion is mainly stimulated by the renin-angiotensin system. Androgen production is stimulated physiologically during early adolescence, probably under the control of ACTH or another central stimulating hormone,

producing 'adrenarche' (see Chapter 4). ACTH, and hence cortisol, is produced in a circadian rhythm, with the highest levels in the early morning. ACTH can also be quickly secreted in times of stress.

a) Failure of aldosterone secretion

Congenital isolated defects of aldosterone biosynthesis with a normal glucocorticoid production are caused by abnormalities in methyloxidases I and II that transform corticosterone into aldosterone. Investigations will reveal hyperkalemia, low-normal or diminished serum sodium levels, metabolic alkalosis and progressive reduction of kidney function, resulting finally in central shock and acidosis. Plasma renin activity is high and aldosterone low. Measurement of plasma corticosterone, 18-OH corticosterone and aldosterone levels along with a urinary steroid profile can demonstrate the precise enzymatic defect. Fludrocortisone acetate is used as replacement therapy (see Chapter 6).

Pseudohypoaldosteronism is caused by a defect of type I aldosterone receptors. The symptoms are the same as those of hypoaldosteronism but aldosterone levels are very high. Administration of fludrocortisone acetate has no effect and high doses of oral sodium chloride are necessary for treatment.

Mineralocorticoid deficiency as part of salt-wasting congenital adrenal hyperplasia is discussed in Chapter 6.

b) Hypoadrenalism

Although hypoadrenalism *per se* does not invariably cause hyponatremia, this is often a major component of the presentation of the causes of hypoadrenocorticism that are listed in **8.13**. Primary hypoadrenocorticism is caused by a disorder in the adrenal itself and manifests itself biochemically by a low serum cortisol level and a high serum ACTH. The secondary forms are associated with low ACTH levels.

Clinical presentation of adrenal salt loss

Infants with aplasia or hypoplasia of the adrenal glands present with:

- Shock, tachycardia, cold and clammy skin, rapid respiration, vascular collapse.
- Hyperpyrexia.
- Cyanosis.
- Skin pigmentation in the later presenting cases.

Depending on the involvement of the zona glomerulosa, salt loss can occur with hyponatremia and hyperkalemia. The differential diagnosis lies between septicemia, intracranial hemorrhage and pulmonary infections. This disorder can be sex-linked recessive or sporadic.

c) Adrenal hemorrhage

This occurs mainly after prolonged labor and/or traumatic deliveries of large infants and occurs more in boys than in girls. Severe clinical signs, similar to those described above, are seen only if the hemorrhages have occurred bilaterally. On physical examination there may be a mass in the flank. On ultrasonography the kidney can be seen to be displaced downward by a hyper-echoic adrenal. Usually calcification is seen after 3–6 weeks. During fulminating infections (particularly meningococcemia, but also during pneumococcal, streptococcal, hemophilus and diphtheric infections) acute adrenal failure can occur. The clinical presentation is with shock and purpura, and if the child dies bilateral adrenal hemorrhage can be seen at autopsy.

d) Chronic hypoadrenocorticism (Addisonism disease)
This is a chronic progressive debilitating illness. Symptoms consist of:
- Weight loss and gastrointestinal complaints (anorexia, nausea, vomiting, diarrhea).
- Cardiovascular problems (hypotension, decrease in heart size).
- Skin hyperpigmentation due to ACTH over-secretion (**1.129**) (particularly on pressure areas and scars (**1.130**), buccal mucosa, axilla, nipples, groin, and the borders of the lips).

Because of the slow progression of the disease diagnosis may be delayed. It is often not suspected until an acute adrenal crisis with dehydration and shock is precipitated by surgery, trauma, or infection. Addisonism disease can be a result of tuberculosis,

AIDS, other rare infections such as coccidiomycosis, blastomycosis and histoplasmosis, amyloidosis and malignant infiltration. It can result from autoimmune disease (which can be due to isolated anti-adrenal antibodies) but is more often as part of the polyglandular syndrome type I (or HAM syndrome) with hypoparathyroidism and moniliasis (**7.3**).

e) Hypoadrenocorticism secondary to insufficient ACTH secretion
This is usually part of multiple pituitary endocrinopathy but can rarely occur as an isolated event. Congenital unresponsiveness to ACTH has also been described. The 3A syndrome of alacrima, achalasia and adrenal hypofunction (**1.143**) is a rare multisystem disorder affecting the autonomic nervous system and is associated with later neurodevelopmental abnormalities.

Diagnostic work-up

Measurements of serum sodium and potassium are obviously necessary, sometimes in association with an estimation of urinary salt excretion. An early morning (0800–0900) serum cortisol measurement allows for simple exclusion of cortical insufficiency. Note that infants up to 3 months of age do not show a circadian rhythm, so that below this age the timing of the sample is not critical and repeated measurements during the day or an ACTH (Synacthen) test will give useful information.

A paired serum ACTH determination will discriminate the primary and secondary forms of hypoadrenalism.

In response to depot Synacthen (see Appendix A) primary defects will show an absent or low serum cortisol response. A sub-optimal rise is also seen in long-standing central defects. To discriminate between pituitary or hypothalamic problems a stimulation test with CRF (corticotrophin releasing factor) can be performed (see Appendix A).

A urinary steroid profile and measurements of plasma adrenal steroids will help discriminate the various biosynthetic disorders. Very long chain fatty acid (VLCFA) levels are abnormal in adrenoleukodystrophy. An auto-antibody screen should be performed along with at least ultrasonic imaging of the adrenals.

Therapy

Acute adrenal insufficiency is treated with fluid and electrolyte replacement (for example 20 ml normal (0.9%) saline per kg body weight in the first hour followed by a regimen tailored to the circulating volume and serum electrolytes). If there is continuing salt loss oral sodium chloride supplements are required (1 g per 10 kg body weight), both for the initial therapy and until stabilized on mineralocorticoid replacement. For this, use deoxycorticosterone

---

Syndromes of hypoadrenocorticism

Primary hypoadrenocorticism
Aplasia or hypoplasia of the adrenals
Adrenal hemorrhage of the newborn
Congenital adrenal hyperplasia caused by:-
   21-hydroxylase deficiency
   11β-hydroxylase deficiency
   17α-hydroxylase deficiency
   3β-hydroxysteroid dehydrogenase deficiency
   lipoid hyperplasia
Adrenal crisis of acute infection
Congenital adrenocortical unresponsiveness to ACTH
Chronic hypoadrenocorticism, (Addisonism)
The 3A syndrome
Primary familial xanthomatosis
Adrenoleukodystrophy
Secondary to insufficient ACTH secretion
Suppression by glucocorticoid therapy
Removal of unilateral secreting adrenal tumours
Starvation, anorexia nervosa
Infants born to mothers treated with steroids
Anencephaly
Secondary to drug therapy - ketoconazole, cyproterone

8.13 Syndromes of hypoadrenocorticism.

acetate (DOCA), at an approximate dose of 2 mg per day intramuscularly, and then change to twice daily 9α-fludrocortisone acetate (0.15–0.25 mg/m^2/24 hours) when the patient is able to take oral fluids. This dose should then be tailored to maintain normal PRA levels and blood pressure.

Hydrocortisone sodium hemisuccinate is given intravenously in a dose of 120 mg/m^2/24 hours or prednisolone 25 mg/m^2/24 hours. This dosage is approximately 10 times the physiological secretion rate. Maintenance therapy consists of hydrocortisone, 12–15 mg/m^2/24 hours, orally every 8 hours commonly divided 2:1:1, to try mimic the natural circadian secretion. The first dose should be given on waking, the second in the early afternoon and the last dose before bedtime. Infants and small toddlers may require a four times a day dose or the use of a pre-bedtime equivalent dose of prednisolone (with a longer half life) to allow safe levels during sleep.

At times of stress the body responds with an increase of ACTH and cortisol production, therefore children with hypoadrenocorticism should be treated at times of fever, minor infections and trauma and even psychological upset, with a double dose of hydrocortisone. For elective surgery, with serious infections or trauma and if a vomiting illness occurs parenteral therapy is required, at 10 times the physiological rate (as at diagnosis). The parents of all hypoadrenocortical children should be instructed how to seek immediate medical help and advice and how to give an initial intramuscular injection of 50–100 mg of hydrocortisone, which may be life saving in some situations.

Hypernatremia due to mineralocorticoid excess
In 11β-hydroxysteroid dehydrogenase (and to a lesser extent in 17α hydroxylase deficiency) there is sufficient accumulation of deoxycorticosterone (DOC) to produce salt retention, hypokalemia and hypertension as well as cortisol deficiency and pseudohermaphroditism (see Chapter 6.)

Overtreatment of 21-hydroxylase deficiency with fludrocortisone will produce salt retention and hypertension.

Other endocrine causes of hypertension
Primary hyperaldosteronism is very rare in childhood, but when it occurs is most likely due to bilateral nodular adrenal hyperplasia or tumor. Plasma expansion, hypernatremia and renin suppression occur. The Cushing syndrome in childhood is often accompanied by hypertension.

Tumors of neural crest origin (pheochromocytoma, neuroblastoma or ganglioneuroma) may produce hypertension secondary to catecholamine excess. They may occur sporadically or in association with neurofibromatosis, von Hippel–Lindau syndrome and MEA 2 and 2b. The hypertension may be intermittent or sustained and accompanied by:
- Headaches
- Pallor and sweating
- Nausea
- Abdominal pain
- Visual loss or diplopia
- Fits

Diagnosis is by determination of plasma catecholamine levels or their urinary metabolites VMA and HVA. The radioisotope MIBG and CT scanning can be used to localize the tumor. Treatment is by surgical resection after combined α- and ß-blockade in a specialist unit.

CALCIUM AND PHOSPHATE

PHYSIOLOGY

The main regulator of calcium and phosphate levels is parathormone (PTH), which is secreted in response to reduced serum calcium concentrations. It increases bone mobilization of calcium and renal calcium reabsorption and (less immediately) it increases calcium absorption in the intestine (through its action on vitamin D metabolism). It also decreases the reabsorption of phosphate from the proximal tubules of the kidney. The effect of PTH on vitamin D metabolism is mediated through an increase of the renal 1-hydroxylase enzyme activity, which transforms 25-(OH) vitamin D into 1,25-(OH)$_2$ vitamin D.

Vitamin D (calciferol) is synthesized from cholesterol in the skin and taken in food and is then transformed to 25-(OH) vitamin D in the liver. In the kidney it is transformed either to the 1,25-(OH)$_2$D (active) or 24,25-(OH)$_2$D (inactive) forms. The activity of 1-hydroxylase is upregulated by PTH and down-regulated by both raised 1,25-(OH)$_2$D and serum phosphate concentrations. It acts on the intestine to increase calcium absorption, mobilizes calcium from bone and reabsorbs calcium in the kidney. Hepatic and renal disease will lead to secondary hypocalcemia by disrupting the synthesis of active vitamin D metabolites and tubular reabsorption of calcium.

The skeleton serves as a store of calcium and phosphate. Parathormone and 1,25-(OH)$_2$D potentiate each other's action on bone resorption. Calcitonin decreases calcium mobilization and increases calcium excretion by the kidney. It is secreted in response to hypercalcemia. It has only a minor role in calcium homeostasis.

INVESTIGATION OF HYPO- OR HYPERCALCEMIA

Serum calcium (Ca) and phosphate (P) measurements should be determined. After the neonatal period, serum calcium levels remain constant throughout childhood (2.1–2.85 mmol/l, 8.4–10.6 mg/dl) whereas serum phosphate is age-dependent, with high levels in early childhood (1.3–2.3 mmol/l, 4–7 mg/dl) decreasing to adult levels (or 0.6–1.5 mmol/l, 2.0–4.6 mg/dl) only after adolescence. Total serum calcium levels should be interpreted in relation to serum albumin and corrected in states of hypo- or hyperalbuminemia by the formula:

Corrected Ca = total Ca mmol/l – (0.25 x albumin g/l) + 1

If abnormalities are detected further investigations are warranted. Intact parathormone, 25(OH)D, 1,25(OH)$_2$D and urine cAMP should be measured. An indirect measure of PTH secretion is an estimation of renal phosphate reabsorption. Renal phosphate excretion occurs mainly by means of failure of reabsorption in the proximal tubule of the kidney. This process is saturable and the ratio of the maximal rate of tubular phosphate reabsorption to the glomerular filtration rate (Tmp/GFR) can be easily determined by simultaneous measurement of fasting urine and serum phosphate and creatinine concentrations. Normal levels of the Tmp/GFR ratio are age dependent, with high values during childhood (1.3–2.6 mmol/l or 4–8 mg/dl) declining to adult levels (0.8–1.4 mmol/l or 2.5–4.2 mg/dl) after the age of 18 years. Parathormone is one of the many factors influencing renal handling of phosphate (in that it resets the Tmp/GFR ratio at a lower level, resulting in increased urinary phosphate excretion and decreased serum phosphate concentrations), accordingly the Tmp/GFR ratio is high in hypoparathyroidism and low in hyperparathyroidism (see Appendix A).

Hypocalcemia

The clinical symptoms and signs of hypocalcemia occur earlier if the calcium level falls rapidly, if serum magnesium is low, if there is an alkalosis, or serum potassium level is high, and comprise:
- Tetany (increased neurological excitability) which can express itself in atypical forms (paresthesia, cramps)
- Stridor, from laryngospasm
- Chvostek's sign (spasm around the mouth and eyes from percussion of the tempero-mandibular branch of the facial nerve)
- Trousseau's sign (spasm of the hand and thumb in response to relative ischemia from a tourniquet)
- Smooth muscle spasm
- Persistent diarrhea
- Seizures
- Extrapyramidal signs due to basal ganglion calcification
- Papilledema
- Raised intracranial pressure
- Psychiatric disorders
- Dermal and dental changes (dry skin, brittle nails, coarse hair)
- Cataracts

Differential diagnosis

A list of causes of hypocalcemia in the neonate and later childhood is shown in **8.14**.

Deficient parathyroid hormone secretion results in hypocalcemia (due to decreased bone mobilisation, renal reabsorption and intestinal absorption). Hyperphosphatemia results from increased renal reabsorption due to inadequate inhibition by PTH. The causes of hypoparathyroidism are given in **8.15**.

Various PTH receptor defects will result in PTH resistant hypocalcemia, pseudohypoparathyroidism (see Chapter 2). Many cases are associated with learning difficulties, short stature, a round face with a short neck, a short fourth metacarpal (see **2.50**) and nodular subcutaneous calcification.

Maternal hyperparathyroidism will cause transient hypocalcemia in the infant due to exposure to a hypercalcemic *in utero* environment and parathormone suppression.

Therapy

Acute

The treatment of tetany, if present, consists of a 10% calcium gluconate infusion at a dosage of 0.20 ml per kg body weight, followed by 1.6 ml per kg (0.36 mmol per kg) over 6-12 hours. Extravasation leads to tissue necrosis (**8.16**, **8.17**) so the solution should be preferably diluted 1:10. If there are no neurological symptoms, oral calcium at 50 mg per kg over 24 hours in 4 divided doses should be used.

Long-term

The aim of therapy is to maintain serum calcium levels at the lower limit of normal. Vitamin D is given as dihydrotachysterol, 1α-hydroxycholecalciferol or 1,25-dihydroxycholecalciferol, usually in combination with calcium supplements (20 mg/kg per day). Overtreatment will result in nephrocalcinosis, therefore regular checks are needed of serum calcium, phosphate and creatinine, as well as urinary calcium excretion over 24 hours. The calcium excretion should not exceed 4 mg per kg (0.1 mmol/kg). Regular renal ultrasonography is also recommended to detect early calcium deposition.

Causes of hypocalcemia

Early neonatal
  Prematurity
  Asphyxia
  Infants of diabetic mothers

Late neonatal
  Hypoparathyroidism – transient or permanent
  High milk phosphate load
  Hypomagnesemia
  Parenteral nutrition
  Exchange transfusions
  Chronic alkalosis or bicarbonate treatment
  Maternal hyperparathyroidism

Childhood
  Vitamin D deficiency (in early or latest stages)
  Vitamin D dependent rickets (types 1 and 2)
  Hypoparathyroidism
  Pseudohypoparathyroidism

8.14 Causes of hypocalcaemia.

Rickets

Rickets is a state of faulty mineralization of bone matrix in a growing child. It may result in hypocalcemia, but the biochemical manifestations are variable. The various causes of rickets are shown in **8.18**.

Clinical signs
- Hard expansion of the bone ends (see **1.40**).
- Skull deformities with frontal bossing and brachycephaly.
- Rachitic rosary (see **1.83**).
- Leg deformities, often with bowing (**8.19, 8.20**).
- Leg pain and refusal to walk.
- Growth retardation (see **2.21**).
- Myopathy.

Radiography
Radiographs of any of the large joints show widening of the growth plate with 'cupping' and irregular concavity at the metaphysis (**8.21**). There may be reduced bone mineralization.

Causes of hypoparathyroidism

Aplasia and hypoplasia
  Isolated – (sporadic, X-linked, autosomal-recessive, maternal I^{131} therapy)
  Dysbranchiogenesis – the DiGeorge syndrome (in association with hypoplastic thymus, cardiac defects and
    abnormalities on chromosome 22q)
  Kenny syndrome – (in association with hypermetropia, short stature and tubular bone stenosis)

Transient hypoparathyroidism
  Transient congenital parathyroid gland dysplasia
  Maternal hyperparathyroidism
  Hypomagnesemia

Polyglandular syndrome type 1 (or HAM syndrome)

Isolated idiopathic hypoparathyroidism

Acquired hypoparathyroidism
  Surgical
  Irradiation
  Infiltration (iron storage in the hemoglobinopathies)

Pseudohypoparathyroidism (Albright's hereditary osteodystrophy)

8.15 Causes of hypoparathyroidism.

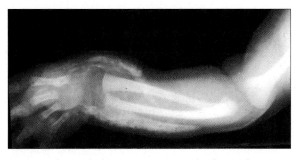

8.16 Radiograph showing extravasated calcium; this required later forearm amputation.

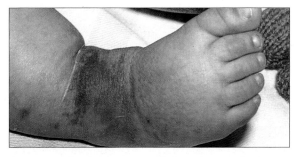

8.17 Superficial tissue necrosis from extravasated calcium that required later plastic surgery.

Therapy and prevention

Simple vitamin D deficient rickets is treated by either 50–150 µg of vitamin D, given daily for two weeks then reduced to 10 µg daily, or by a single intramuscular dose of 15,000 µg of vitamin D (ergocalciferol).

Vitamin D-dependent rickets type 1 (secondary to a deficiency or absence of 1α-hydroxylating enzyme) is treated with calcitriol 0.25–2 µg/24 hours. Vitamin D-dependent rickets type 2 (severe unresponsiveness to 1,25-(OH)$_2$D) can be treated with large doses of calcitriol.

Hypophosphatemic rickets is treated with oral phosphate supplements coupled with calcitriol. There is some evidence that growth hormone will improve the tubular phosphate loss and also improve the rate of growth.

Osteoporosis

Juvenile idiopathic osteoporosis (**8.22**) is a condition of unknown cause that produces bone pain and fractures in the prepubertal child, but seems distinct from osteogenesis imperfecta. It remits after several

The forms of rickets

	Ca	P	PTH
Vitamin D deficiency			
Stage 1, early	Low	Normal	Normal
Stage 2	Normal	Low	High
Stage 3, late	Low	Low	Low
X–linked hypo-phosphatemia	Normal	Very low	Normal
Type 1 Vitamin D dependent	Low	Low	High
Type 2 Vitamin D dependent + alopecia.	Low	Low	High

8.18 The forms of rickets.

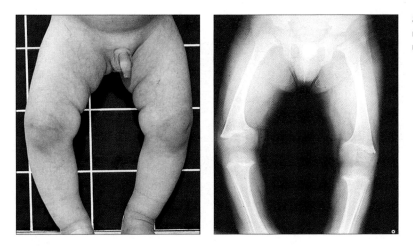

8.19, 8.20 Vitamin D deficient rickets, external appearance and radiograph.

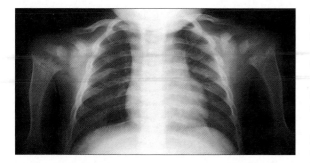

8.21 Chest radiograph showing widened epiphyses, cupping of the metaphyses and abnormal bone formation in hypophosphatemic rickets.

years but can leave residual deformity and short stature. The serum calcium levels are low whilst the disease is active.

Any causes of pubertal delay (see Chapter 5) can produce under-mineralization of the skeleton, detectable on estimation of bone mineral density, that tends to be more severe with later presentation. Whether this produces clinically important later effects is unknown, but spontaneous fractures have been reported in adults with the Ullrich–Turner syndrome. The Cushing syndrome can produce vertebral collapse and permanent stunting due to low mineral density.

Hypercalcemia

The clinical symptoms and signs of hypercalcemia are:
- Weakness
- Vomiting and constipation
- Polyuria and polydipsia

Nephrocalcinosis may occur leading to renal failure and secondary hypertension.

Hyperparathyroidism may be caused by an adenoma or general hyperplasia of the glands and is rare in childhood. Adenomas are sporadic but hyperplasia may be familial and associated with MEA 1 or 2.

Vitamin D intoxication and malignancy may also cause hypercalcemia.

In infancy transient idiopathic hypercalcemia is associated with characteristic facial features (**8.23**) and cardiovascular defects (Williams syndrome).

An infantile form of severe primary hyperparathyroidism due to hyperplasia of the glands may occur. It presents with marked hypotonia, feeding problems, chest deformity and respiratory distress. It may be familial or sporadic and usually the cause is unknown. It is severe enough to warrant emergency total parathyroidectomy. Maternal hypocalcemia due to hypoparathyroidism or other causes will result in transient reactive hypercalcemia after birth. Phosphate depletion in the light-for-dates or preterm infant may also cause infantile hypercalcemia.

GLUCOSE

Glucose input from the diet and tissue stores is balanced against utilization by the tissues. Pancreatic endocrine secretion of insulin, as well as glucagon, somatostatin and pancreatic polypeptide, is modulated by nutrient levels (glucose and amino acids), autonomic neural input and by paracrine influences. Insulin will act to move glucose into fat and muscle, promote liver glycogen synthesis and has an anabolic action on muscle protein synthesis. These actions result in a lowering of glucose, ketone body, free fatty acid and branch chain amino acid levels. Glucagon rises at the expense of insulin during periods of starvation, possibly in part modulated by the effects of pancreatic somatostatin. As glucose concentrations fall there is a reciprocal rise in the extra-pancreatic counter-regulatory hormones cortisol, growth hormone and adrenaline that act in various ways to stabilize blood glucose levels. Growth is adaptively

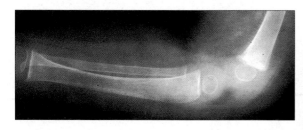

8.22 Juvenile idiopathic osteoporosis.

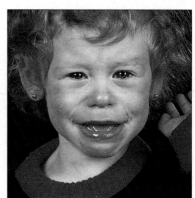

8.23 The Williams syndrome. Note abnormal mid-face and wide-open mouth. The iris has a stellate appearance (not shown), the voice is hoarse and there may be hyperacusis.

inhibited, despite the rise in GH, by a rise in levels of IGFBP-1 and thus reduced growth factor availability. It follows that any relative excess of insulin or lack of counter-regulatory hormones will tend to produce hypoglycemia. Insulin deficiency (usually seen in type 1 insulin dependent diabetes mellitus) or insulin resistance (seen much more rarely in childhood as MODY (maturity onset diabetes of youth) or with other syndromic associations) will produce hyperglycemia. Cortisol excess, either iatrogenic or as part of the Cushing syndrome, will also produce hyperglycemia (as can iatrogenic overdosage with GH in rare clinical situations).

HYPOGLYCEMIA

Hypoglycemia triggers a set of counter-regulatory and neuro-behavioral responses. The blood glucose level that achieves these effects is to an extent age, disease and situation dependent but may approximately be taken as <2.2 mmol/l (40 mg/dl) in the older child or adult and < 2.8 (50 mg/dl) in the neonate, although levels less than 3.5 mmol/l (62 mg/dl) may be of concern in the sick, premature infant.

Hypoglycemia itself modifies especially the metabolic responses to subsequent episodes of low blood sugar, both in the long- and short-term, and there may also be changes with disease duration and activity. Some metabolic disorders that cause hypoglycemia also affect normal counter-regulation, further complicating the predictability of symptoms.

Clinical presentation
The presenting features of hypoglycemia in childhood are:
- Pallor and sweating
- Confusion and irritability, proceeding to loss of consciousness
- Hunger, abdominal pain or nausea
- Convulsions

In the neonate, additionally:
- Jitteriness
- Hypotonia
- Hypothermia
- Apnea and oxygen desaturation
- Tachypnea

Differential diagnosis
In the neonate hyperinsulinism caused by diabetes in the mother or by pancreatic endocrine dysregulation syndrome could be associated with macrosomia (see **3.22, 3.24**). Neonatal hyperinsulinism can also be secondary to hydrops fetalis. Premature babies and small-for-dates infants (see **2.16**) have decreased energy stores in the presence of increased utilization.

The Beckwith–Wiedemann or EMG syndrome (exomphalos, macroglossia, gigantism) (see **3.9–3.11**) may be associated with an abnormality of chromosome 11 in a proportion of patients and there is a risk of Wilms tumor and other malignancies (see Chapter 3).

Panhypopituitarism in the male neonate may be evident from micropenis or cryptorchidism (see **6.9, 6.10**). Although the importance of growth hormone as a counter-regulatory hormone wanes after the first year of life, there is genetic variability in mechanisms of glucose homeostasis and hypoglycemia may be a presenting feature of isolated GHD or hypopituitarism even in the older child (who will also manifest a poor rate of growth, short stature or hypogonadism).

There may be hepatomegaly associated with the glycogen storage disorders both in the neonatal period and at later presentation (see **2.24, 2.25**). Fatty acid oxidation disorders, galactosemia and some other metabolic disorders will produce hypoglycemia as a consequence of decreased production of glucose, as will severe liver disease. Alcohol ingestion in childhood may be associated with severe hypoglycemia.

Pancreatic adenomas can occur in later childhood *de novo* or as part of MEN 1.

Diagnostic work-up
At the time of hypoglycemia (which may need to be induced by starvation in some carefully supervised situations in specialized centers) blood should be obtained to allow comparison of the low blood glucose levels to insulin, cortisol and growth hormone. Also estimate branched chain amino acids, hydroxy-butarate, lactate and free fatty acids. The first urine passed after the episode should be analyzed for dicarboxylic acids, glycine conjugates, organic acids and acylcarnitine. If there is any possibility of factitious hypoglycemia then assay C-peptide levels (which will be low at the same time as a raised insulin if this is being administered by a carer) and for alcohol, salicylate or oral hypoglycemic agents such as sulfonylurea.

Hypoglycemia can be broadly classified as ketotic or non-ketotic and a summary of the interpretation of these investigations is given in **8.24**.

Therapy
Hypoglycemia should be treated with oral carbohydrate if possible. Some situations will respond to glucagon 0.5–1 mg intramuscularly, although this requires available hepatic glycogen stores in order to be effective. Severe symptomatic hypoglycemia should be treated using an infusion of 2 ml/kg 10% dextrose over 3 minutes followed by 0.1 ml/kg/minute adjusted to keep the blood sugar between 5–8 mmol/l (90–140 mg/dl). Stronger glucose solutions should almost never be used as there is a risk of hyperosmolar damage to the CNS.

HYPERGLYCEMIA AND GLYCOSURIA

Symptomatic hyperglycemia in childhood is almost always associated with type 1 insulin dependent diabetes mellitus (IDDM). The presenting features are:
- Polyuria.
- Polydipsia.
- Weight loss.
- Diabetic ketoacidosis.
- Candidiasis or recurrent staphylococcal skin infections.

It is not infrequently diagnosed by the serendipitous demonstration of glycosuria, or by screening in children with previously affected relatives.

Clinically significant complications of diabetes are rare in childhood although joint stiffness (see **1.19**) and microalbuminuria may be detected on screening.

Diabetic retinopathy (**8.25**) rarely may be present at, or soon after, presentation in some individuals, presumably representing an inherent genetic susceptibility to this complication. All patients should have their dilated fundi regularly examined.

There is an increased incidence of IDDM in the Klinefelter syndrome and a number of non-chromosomal syndromes. True IDDM may occur in the neonatal period (**8.26**) but there is also a syndrome of transient neonatal diabetes that is characterized by the early onset of glycosuria and wasting and extreme sensitivity to exogenous insulin. The illness is of unknown etiology but remits spontaneously after a few weeks or months.

Insulin resistance may be a feature of several dysmorphic conditions including the Ullrich–Turner, Bardet–Biedl and Prader–Labhart–Willi syndromes

---

Investigation of hypoglycemia

Ketosis plus fatty acid elevation =
Growth hormone deficiency
    (In the neonate the GH response to hypoglycemia is variable and may require later provocation testing to confirm. Treatment with GH and restoration of normoglycemia is an initial pragmatic approach)
Cortisol deficiency, confirmed by low cortisol.

No Ketosis plus low fatty acids =
Hyperinsulinism – confirm with detectable (not necessarily absolutely raised) insulin level
Sometimes panhypopituitarism in the neonate

No Ketosis plus raised fatty acids = Fatty acid oxidation defects

Lactate raised = Inborn error of metabolism

C peptide low whilst insulin high = Factitious administration of insulin

8.24 Investigation of hypoglycaemia.

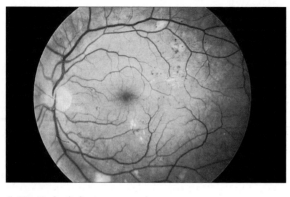

8.25 Early diabetic retinopathy.

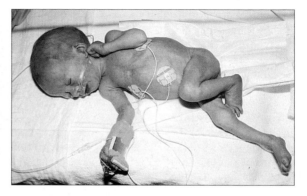

8.26 Neonatal diabetes mellitus – presenting as gross failure to thrive.

(see Chapter 2). Insulin resistance is also seen in association with the leprechaun syndrome (see **1.117**), with acanthosis nigricans (see **1.131, 1.132**) and other syndromes of insulin resistance. The possibility now exists of treating this form of resistance with recombinant IGF-1.

Maturity onset diabetes of youth (MODY) is rare but characterized by the onset, at less than 25 years of age, of the autosomal dominant inheritance of a primary defect in insulin secretion. It is due to several different mutations at chromosomes 7q and 20q.

The management of diabetes in childhood should involve a multi-disciplinary team-based approach to treat and support the child and family and to try to prevent the later onset of complications by optimizing glucose control. The interested reader is referred to one of the texts devoted to this topic cited on page 143.

SCREENING SURVIVORS OF PEDIATRIC MALIGNANCY

The success of the treatments for various childhood malignancies means that increasing numbers of long-term survivors require follow-up. It is estimated that by the year 2000 almost 1 in a thousand of the young adult population will fall into this category.

The cost of the cure is related to the chemo- and radiotherapy received during initial treatment. Many survivors will have short stature and endocrine dysfunction (see **2.47**). The exact nature of the later endocrine and growth inhibiting effects will depend on the nature, dosage, age of administration and sex of the patient. The relative contributions of drug and radiation induced effects are still far from clear. Only active surveillance for the development of these problems at an early stage will allow for early detection and treatment before avoidable morbidity occurs.

An outline of the endocrine and other problems that will require prospective surveillance in these survivors is given in **8.27**.

ARTEFACTUAL ENDOCRINOPATHIES

Any laboratory assay has an inbuilt error of estimation. If the results obtained on testing do not agree with the clinical picture it is always wise to raise the possibility of laboratory error or repeat the estimation. Many diagnostic 'kits' come with inappropriate reference ranges for children and it is wise to establish local experience and 'normal' values with an assay before routine use. It should be remembered that 'normality' is usually defined as a value ±2 stan-

dard deviations from the mean and some outliers will, by definition, be healthy individuals.

'Adequate' responses to stimulation tests (especially with respect to growth hormone) are often defined in an arbitrary way and change with availability of treatment and medical practice. Apparent lack of response may reflect poor investigative methodology more than pathology. Failure to appreciate changes in hormone levels with time of day, age, weight or surface area will also lead to confusion. Some international hormone standards measured in units referable to a biological standard also change from time to time and require revision of normal values.

There are some apparent endocrine abnormalities that are due to more predictable laboratory artefacts or to biological or induced variation in binding protein levels or hormone metabolism. These are briefly discussed below.

DRUGS AND DIET

Many drugs will induce liver enzymes and hence increase hormone clearance or binding protein levels and thus interfere with total hormone estimations. Alkaline phosphatase levels may also be altered. The H_2 histamine blockers, such as cimetidine, interfere with the measurement of serum calcium. *It is thus essential that a drug history is provided to the laboratory.* Food with a high vanilla content and a number of drugs will interfere with urinary estimation of VMA and HVA.

HYPERLIPIDEMIA

Hyperlipidemia (**8.28**) may be seen in diabetic ketoacidosis and interferes with some laboratory electrochemical methods of sodium analysis to produce apparent hyponatremia.

BINDING PROTEIN ABNORMALITIES

Cortisol, testosterone and thyroxine are bound to specific circulating binding proteins (BPs) as well as serum albumen. Measurement of total levels of these hormones will therefore overestimate biological activity in states of binding protein excess and underestimate activity with low BP levels. General states of protein loss, such as nephrotic syndrome, or decreased production, as in cirrhosis of the liver, will affect all the BPs.

Corticosteroid binding globulin (CBG) levels are elevated by estrogen, producing high levels of

Surveillance in survivors of childhood malignancy

Growth impairment

1. Proportionate loss (GHD)	Cranial irradiation – onset of GHD in proportion to the dose and younger age of treatment
2. ± Short spine (GHD + spinal damage)	Spinal irradiation; abdominal or thoracic irradiation; Total body irradiation (TBI)
(?epiphyseal toxicity)	? Chemotherapy including 6-Mercaptopurine

Gonadal Dysfunction

Females

Primary ovarian failure	TBI, abdominal irradiation
Premature ovarian failure	Cyclophosphamide
Central precocious puberty (contributes to height loss)	Low dose cranial irradiation (18–24 Gy)

Males

Testicular failure (Leydig cells + germinal epithelium)	Direct irradiation (as in some ALL treatment regimens and testicular tumors; TBI) Scatter irradiation from abdominal tumor
Infertility (germinal epithelium)	Chemotherapy – especially cyclophosphamide,vinblastine and procarbazine. Direct irradiation

Thyroid Dysfunction

Thyroid failure	Direct irradiation - (Hodgkin's disease),or as part of craniospinal irradiation and TBI. TSH lack secondary to cranial irradiation
Thyroid malignancy	In proportion to the dose received by gland, special risk if TSH is elevated.

Adrenal Insufficiency

Hypocortisolemia	Rare, but can occur after high dose irradiation for cranial tumors

Posterior Pituitary

Diabetes Insipidus	Rare – usually after neurosurgery for cranial tumors

Other

Renal damage and hypertension	Chemotherapy, direct irradiation
Cardiac toxicity	Anthracycline chemotherapy, ± radiation damage
CNS damage	Irradiation in proportion to the dose received, more with early age of therapy. Direct trauma from surgery
Vision	Cataracts from irradiation. Damage to optic tracts from irradiation and surgery
Second malignancies	Skin and soft tissue in irradiation field. 2nd tumors with alkylating agents or genetic predisposition
Dental caries	Most chemotherapy

8.27 Surveillance in survivors of childhood malignancy.

measured cortisol in pregnancy and with estrogen therapy. Low levels are seen in hypothyroidism and obesity. Genetic disorders producing high and low CBG levels have been described.

Testosterone binding protein (or sex hormone binding globulin, SHBG) levels are increased in androgen deficiency states, with estrogen treatment and in thyrotoxicosis. Levels are low in obesity, hypothyroidism, the Cushing syndrome and after androgen treatment. Again hereditary abnormalities of production have been described. Estrogen largely circulates bound to albumen and will therefore appear decreased in nephrotic syndrome.

Probably the most clinically important binding protein considerations are in relation to the assessment of thyroid function. It is now common to be able to assay free hormone activity directly, avoiding some of these difficulties. A summary of diseases and drugs that will interfere with the interpretation of thyroid function tests is shown in (**8.29**).

Carbohydrate Deficient Glycoprotein syndrome is a rare generalized disorder of serum glycoproteins that is associated with developmental delay, organ failure and adult hypogonadism. There is a deficiency of TBG, CBG and SHBG and consequently low levels of these hormones on total assay. Associated abnormalities of unbound LH, FSH, prolactin and GH have also been described in this complex syndrome.

MATERNAL HORMONE ABNORMALITIES IN PREGNANCY DUE TO FETAL EFFECTS

The feto-placental axis is 'added-on' to the maternal hormone system through pregnancy. The fetal adrenal cortex plays an important role in producing hormones which appear to be vital for placental function. In particular, dehydroepiandrosterone (DHEA) is produced in large quantities, and further processed to estrogens in the placenta. Maternal urinary excretion of estriol (E3) in particular provides useful information about the fetal pituitary-adrenal axis. Low levels of estriol indicate fetal adrenal insufficiency, either primary or secondary. (Undetectable maternal estriols are found in placental sulfatase deficiency producing a syndrome of post-maturity and congenital ichthyosis [see **1.142**]). Maternal virilization has been reported as a consequence of fetal p450 aromatase deficiency (converting testosterone to estradiol) with the later delivery of an female pseudo-hermaphroditic infant.

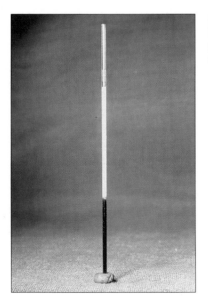

8.28 Gross hyperlipidemia in glycogen storage disease type 1.

Induced abnormalities of thyroid function tests				
	T4	**FT4**	**T3**	**TSH**
Renal failure	↓	↓	↓	→
Hepatic failure	↓	↓	↓	→↑
Estrogen Rx	↑	→	→↑	→
Propanolol Rx	↑	→	↑	→
Epilepsy Rx	↓	→	↓	→
High dose steroids	↓	→	↓	→
GH Rx	↓	→	↑	↑
HCG Rx or choriocarcinoma	↑	↑	↑	↓

8.29 Induced abnormalities of thyroid function tests.

Suggested Reference Texts

Becker KL (Ed). *Principles and Practice of Endocrinology and Metabolism*, 2nd Edn, 1995. Lippincott, Philadelphia, USA.

Beighton P. *Inherited Disorders of the Skeleton*, 1988. Churchill Livingstone, Edinburgh, UK.

Besser GM, Thorner MO. *Clinical Endocrinology*, 1994. Wolfe, London, UK.

Brook CDG (Ed). *Clinical Paediatric Endocrinology*, 3rd Edn, 1995. Blackwell Scientific, Oxford, UK.

Hughes IA. *Handbook of Endocrine Investigations in Children*, 1989. Wright, London, UK.

Kappy MS, Blizzard RM, Migeon CJ (Eds). *Wilkins. The Diagnosis and Treatment of Endocrine Disorders in Childhood and Adolescence*, 1994. Charles Thomas, Springfield, USA.

Kelnar C (Ed). *Childhood Diabetes*, 1994. Chapman and Hall, London, UK.

Lifshitz F (Ed). *Pediatric Endocrinology: A Clinical Guide*, 1990. Dekker, USA.

Ranke MB (Ed). *Functional Endocrine Diagnostics in Children and Adolescents*, 1992. JJ Verlag, Mannheim, Germany.

Winter RM, Baraitser M. *Multiple Congenital Abnormalities, a diagnostic compendium*, 1991. Chapman and Hall, London, UK. (Also available as computerized London Dysmorphology Database.)

Appendices

Appendix A

Tests of Endocrine Function

INTRODUCTORY NOTES

These protocols are included for general guidance only. They were designed for use in a specialist children's endocrine unit and may not always be applicable elsewhere. It is the responsibility of clinicians performing the tests to ensure that correct local procedures are followed, particularly in relation to the administration of drugs, patient safety and comfort.

Further information on dynamic testing can be obtained from one of the texts cited on page 143.

COMBINED ANTERIOR PITUITARY FUNCTION TEST

PRINCIPLE

A combined provocation test is used to test for adequate excretion of GH, TSH, LH and FSH. The 'gold standard' test is still the insulin tolerance test + TRH + GnRH test, which has the advantage of allowing the assessment of ACTH secretion in response to hypoglycemia in a more predictable manner than with clonidine. However, this test has led to death in some circumstances and it should remain confined to experienced units, who will already have an established protocol. It will not therefore be described in this section.

MATERIALS REQUIRED
Pharmaceutical:
- Clonidine. TRH and LHRH (separately or combined in a single ampoule).
- Depot testosterone (for boys of TW2 bone age greater than 10 years).

Other:
- Lithium heparin containers.

APPROXIMATE LENGTH OF TEST
Three hours excluding any overnight preparation.

PATIENT PREPARATION
The exact procedure employed in males depends upon the age of the patient. If older than 10 years but with no signs of endogenous sexual development then consideration should be given to prior priming with sex steroids as there is good evidence that false positive results will result in the relatively hypogonadotropic milieu of delayed puberty. Sex steroid priming is achieved by giving 100 mg depot testosterone esters i.m. 3–5 days before the test. There is no evidence that priming of females is required.

The patient is fasted overnight prior to the test. Venous access is secured and fixed into position along with a three-way stopcock for the duration of the test. The line is kept patent with heparinized saline.

Clonidine may make the subject nauseated, dizzy and hypotensive. TRH and GnRH can produce flushing and a metallic taste in the mouth. The subject must be fully recovered and have taken a meal before discharge home.

PROCEDURE
Oral clonidine (150 µg per m^2) is given at time 0.

The standard dose of TRH is 5–7 µg/kg (up to 200 µg) and of GnRH 2.5 µg/kg (up to 100 µg) injected over 2 minutes at time 0, immediately after the clonidine has been taken.

SAMPLES REQUIRED
Blood is collected at each time point according to schedule **A1** on p. 146. The volume required will vary according to local laboratory needs. The time of collection of the samples should be strictly recorded.

INTERPRETATION OF RESULTS

Growth hormone

Adequate secretion — more than 20 IU/l.

As discussed in Chapter 2 this level is arbitrary, and has tended to increase over time. Certainly levels of 10 IU/l or less are indicative of more severe deficiency than intermediate levels.

TSH

Hypopituitary

- all levels within normal basal range, **and**
- an increase to peak level of less than 5 IU/l (when basal level was less than 2 IU/l), **or**
- an increase to peak level of less than threefold basal (when basal level was greater than 2 IU/l)

Hypothalamic

- level at 20 min more than five times the upper limit of the normal basal range, **or**
- level at 20 min less than level at 60 min (when both levels are above the normal basal range), with a slow fall from this peak if a 120 minute sample is analyzed.

Normal

- Results which are neither hypopituitary nor hypothalamic.

FSH and LH

Normal pubertal response – peak levels are more than threefold greater than basal. This must be interpreted in relation to bone age (see below) and physical maturation.

Prolactin

Prolactin is released in response to TRH. A similar rising 'hypothalamic pattern' may be seen. Basal levels should be interpreted in relation to the reference range. Inappropriate elevation may be seen secondary to compression of the pituitary stalk or with prolactinomas.

Cortisol

Cortisol may rise in response to clonidine administration, reflecting an intact hypothalamo-pituitary axis. If started after an overnight fast the basal level should be high in relation to a previously collected midnight or late evening sample, thus proving an intact circadian rhythm.

Testosterone, estradiol

Normal – basal levels within the age appropriate reference ranges (see below).

Other tests of GH release

A safe alternative to clonidine is to use arginine monohydrochloride, 12.5% solution, 0.5 g/kg infused over 30 minutes with blood taken at –30 minutes in addition to those samples described above.

Glucagon, GHRH, L-Dopa and metaclopramide have all at some time been used as GH secretagogues.

Schedule of sample collection for Combined Anterior Pituitary Function Test

TIME (min)	GH	FT4	TSH	FSH & LH	Cortisol	Testosterone and E2	Prolactin
0	+	+	+	+	+	+	+
			Give clonidine, TRH & GnRH				
20	+	–	+	+	+	–	+
60	+	–	+	+	+	–	+
90	+	–	–	–	+	–	–
120	+	–	±	–	+	–	–
150	+	–	–	–	+	–	–

A1 Schedule of sample collection for Combined Anterior Pituitary Function Test.

GROWTH HORMONE SUPPRESSION TEST

PRINCIPLE
Glucose, given as in an oral glucose tolerance test (GTT), will suppress GH production except in situations of pituitary overproduction.

MATERIALS REQUIRED
Pharmaceutical:
- Oral glucose solution.

Other:
- Fluoride oxalate and heparinized containers.

APPROXIMATE LENGTH OF TEST
Three hours excluding overnight fast.

PATIENT PREPARATION
The patient should be admitted after an overnight fast. Venous access should be secured.

PROCEDURE
Samples for glucose and GH are collected at time zero and then 1.75 g/kg of glucose is administered orally (maximum dose 75g). Blood is drawn at 30, 60, 90 and 120 minutes. Test any urine passed for the presence of glucose.

INTERPRETATION OF RESULTS
Basal GH should be less than 10 IU/l. It should fall to <2 IU/l through the test. Failure to suppress GH levels and an abnormal glucose response (true blood sugar > than 10 mmol/l (182 mg/dl) = frank diabetes, >6.7 mmol/l (122 mg/dl) = impaired glucose tolerance) is indicative of a pituitary adenoma.

GH may fail to suppress in chronic severe anemia, hepatic cirrhosis, porphyria and malnutrition.

ORAL GLUCOSE TOLERANCE TEST

Glucose tolerance tests are much less commonly required in children than in adults. Children usually develop diabetes mellitus rapidly and present as clearly diabetic. The diagnosis can almost always be made by a random fasting plasma glucose. The procedure is the same as outlined above for a GH suppression test (omitting the measurement of GH but sometimes including the simultaneous assay of insulin).

INTRAVENOUS GLUCOSE TOLERANCE TEST

PRINCIPLE
An intravenous glucose tolerance eliminates gastrointestinal factors which can affect the oral test. It allows calculation of a disappearance rate for circulating glucose which is related to insulin status. The test is only rarely performed.

MATERIALS REQUIRED
Pharmaceutical:
- D-glucose as a 50% solution w/v in water.

Other:
- Fluoride oxalate bottles for blood.

APPROXIMATE LENGTH OF TEST
1.5 hours plus overnight fast.

PATIENT PREPARATION
Fast patient overnight.

SAMPLES REQUIRED
Blood in fluoride oxalate tubes at each time point.

PROCEDURE
Glucose is given i.v. as a 25% solution at a dose of 0.5 g/kg body weight over 5 minutes A stopwatch is started when half the dose has been given. Blood samples are collected at exactly 5, 10, 20, 30 and 60 minutes. All urine passed over two hours is tested for glucose.

INTERPRETATION OF RESULTS
Blood glucose results versus time are plotted on semi-logarithmic graph paper to calculate the half life. The disappearance constant, k, is calculated:

$$k\ (\%\ \text{per minute}\ ) = \frac{0.693 \times 100}{\text{half life}}$$

Disappearance rates are normally 1 - 3 % . They are reduced in diabetes and increased in hyperinsulinism.

WATER DEPRIVATION (URINE CONCENTRATION) AND DDAVP STIMULATION TESTS

PRINCIPLE

Fluid intake is restricted and urine osmolality measured to assess renal concentrating ability. DDAVP may be administered to distinguish renal tubular from posterior pituitary dysfunction.

MATERIALS REQUIRED

Pharmaceutical:
• DDAVP (1-deamino-8-D-arginine vasopressin).
Other:
• Universal containers for urine.
• Lithium heparin tubes for blood.

APPROXIMATE LENGTH OF TEST

1-2 days.

PATIENT PREPARATION

The patient is weighed before and periodically during the test. The frequency of weighing depends on the age of the child and suspected disorder. It should not be less frequently than four hourly and may have to be hourly or even half hourly in suspected nephrogenic diabetes insipidus. Calculate 5% of the body weight, subtract it from the starting weight and discontinue the test if the patient's weight falls below this level. Terminate the test at any time if there are clinical signs of serious dehydration.

SAMPLES REQUIRED

Lithium heparin blood samples for sodium and serum osmolality. Urine container for osmolality. Note time of collection on tubes.

PROCEDURE: FLUID DEPRIVATION TEST
Day 1

Normal diet and fluid intake. Send each specimen of urine passed for measurement of volume and osmolality – at least every 4 hours. Note the collection time on the container. If the osmolality of any urine is greater than 700 mmol/l (mOsmol/l), no further testing is required.

Day 2

At 0830 give a normal feed. Weigh the patient. Allow no more food or fluid. Collect blood samples for osmolality and sodium. Collect all urine passed and send immediately to the laboratory for the measurement of volume and osmolality as before.

Collect blood for osmolality and sodium at least four hourly. Terminate the test as soon as any urine osmolality is greater than 700 mmol/l or if there are clinical signs of significant dehydration.

The length of the test depends upon the age of the child and clinical response to dehydration. Careful observation of the child is required throughout the test.

INTERPRETATION OF RESULTS

If any urine sample has an osmolality greater than 700 mmol/l (mOsmol/l), concentrating ability is adequate and the test should be terminated.

If there has been inadequate urinary concentration, proceed to a DDAVP test.

PROCEDURE: DDAVP TEST

The patient is allowed to eat and drink normally (restrict infants to half normal fluid intake to prevent over-hydration). DDAVP is given i.m. at a dose of 0.125 µg for children and one tenth of this for infants (who may be extremely sensitive to DDAVP in the presence of congenital DI). Alternatively intranasal DDAVP can be used at approximately 10 times the i.m. dose.

INTERPRETATION OF RESULTS

If adequate concentration is achieved after DDAVP this suggests satisfactory renal concentrating ability but an inadequate secretion of posterior pituitary AVP (central DI). If there is inadequate concentrating ability after DDAVP renal unresponsiveness to AVP (nephrogenic DI) is demonstrated.

SYNACTHEN TEST

PRINCIPLE

A synthetic form of ACTH is given to test the responsiveness of the adrenal cortex by production of cortisol. Estimation of intermediary compounds, i.e. 17α-hydroxy-progesterone, can give information about biosynthetic defects, such as atypical 21-hydroxylase deficiency.

MATERIALS REQUIRED

Pharmaceutical:
• Synacthen – tetracosactrin acetate.
Other:
• Lithium heparin tubes for blood.

APPROXIMATE LENGTH OF TEST
1.5 hours plus prior overnight stay.

PATIENT PREPARATION
Blood should have been collected at midnight prior to the test.

Anaphylaxis can occur rarely in response to Synacthen and so a supply of emergency drugs should be available and the patient carefully supervised.

SAMPLES REQUIRED
Lithium heparin blood at each time point for cortisol.

PROCEDURE
Give Synacthen i.m. as follows:
Collect blood 30 before and 60 minutes after dose.

AGE	DOSE
0–6 months	62.5 µg
6 months–2 years	125 µg
over 2 years	250 µg

INTERPRETATION OF RESULTS
The midnight and pre-dose cortisols should show a normal diurnal variation (midnight up to 280 nmol/l (10 µg/dl) 0830 am pre-dose 120–660 nmol/l (4.3–23.5 µg/dl).

The normal response to Synacthen is a rise of at least 280 nmol/l (10 µg/dl) to a peak of at least 700 nmol/l (25 µg/dl). Inadequate response indicates impaired adrenal cortical function.

A rise in 17α-hydroxyprogesterone to levels >10 nmol/l (5 µg/l) is seen in atypical 21-hydroxylase deficiency.

DEXAMETHASONE SUPPRESSION TESTS

PRINCIPLE
Dexamethasone is a potent steroid that will suppress ACTH secretion, and hence cortisol in the normal situation.

MATERIALS REQUIRED
Pharmaceutical:
- Dexamethasone.

Other:
- Lithium heparin tubes for blood.

APPROXIMATE LENGTH OF TEST
1 day for overnight test, 5 days for the high dose test.

SAMPLES REQUIRED
Lithium heparin blood at each time point for cortisol and ACTH, urine containers for free cortisol estimation and urinary steroid profile.

PROCEDURE AND INTERPRETATION OF RESULTS
Measure basal cortisol and ACTH:

If both are raised administer oral dexamethasone, 1.0 mg per 1.7 m² at 2300 hours. Determine serum cortisol at 0800-0900 hours the following morning. The morning cortisol should be lower than 50 nmol/l (1.8 µg/dl) or at least 50% of the pre-test morning cortisol.

If the ACTH is undetectable and there is hypercortisolemia, then an adrenal cause is proven and no further tests are required.

If the ACTH is detectable/raised and there is failure of suppression of cortisol in response to the overnight test then administer dexamethasone in a dosage of 0.5 mg per m² four times a day for 2 days and repeat the blood estimations. Then continue with dexamethasone 2.0 mg per m² four times a day for another 2 days.

Collect 24 hour urine samples each day for free urinary free cortisol and steroid profile.

If cortisol excretion is not suppressed by the low dose of dexamethasone, some form of the Cushing syndrome is virtually certain. If there is some suppression on the higher dosage, pituitary Cushing disease is most likely, whilst a lack of any suppression indicates an adrenal tumor.

INVESTIGATION OF HYPOGLYCEMIA IN CHILDREN

PRINCIPLE
Hypoglycemia has a wide variety of causes in children (see Chapter 8). These include various metabolic problems in which hypoglycemic episodes occur intermittently. In order to overcome this difficulty in investigation, a suitable approach is the measurement of the intermediary metabolites directly involved in glucose homeostasis after a prolonged,

supervised fast (12–24 hours depending on age), or during an actual hypoglycemic attack.

MATERIALS REQUIRED
Lithium heparin and fluoride oxalate containers for blood; urine containers.

APPROXIMATE LENGTH OF TEST
Up to 24 hours.

PATIENT PREPARATION
For a prolonged fast, start the test between 16.00 and 21.00 and take samples at 09.00 and 12.00 or 16.00 the following day. The patient can be given water to drink during this time. It is advisable to check the plasma glucose regularly and if symptoms of hypoglycemia occur, either by laboratory assay or on the ward by a reliable bedside method, then terminate the test and treat with oral glucose or i.v.

2 ml/kg 10% dextrose over 3 minutes followed by an infusion of 0.1 ml/kg/minute to keep the blood sugar between 5 and 8 mmol/l (90–144 mg/dl). If hypopituitarism is suspected also give 100 mg of hydrocortisone intravenously.

In infancy it is advisable to start the fast in daylight hours.

SAMPLES REQUIRED
- Fluoride tube: glucose, lactate, alanine, free fatty acids, β-hydroxybutarate and carnitine.
- Heparinized blood: cortisol, GH and insulin (plasma should be separated from cells promptly and stored at -20°C).
- Urine sample as soon as possible after hypoglycemia for organic acids and acylcarnitines.

INTERPRETATION
See Chapter 8.

PTH INFUSION TEST (cAMP EXCRETION)

PRINCIPLE
The excretion of cyclic adenosine monophosphate (cAMP) in urine in response to infused parathyroid hormone (PTH) can be used to discriminate between types of hypoparathyroidism.

MATERIALS REQUIRED
Pharmaceutical:
- PTH for injection 200 iu.
- Human serum albumin (2.5 ml).
- Normal (0.9%) saline (60 ml).

For infusion, dissolve the contents of the PTH ampoule in the albumin which is then added to the saline.
Other:
- Plain containers for PTH.
- Lithium heparin containers for calcium, creatinine, phosphate and sodium assays.

APPROXIMATE LENGTH OF TEST
Three hours excluding overnight fast.

PATIENT PREPARATION
The patient is fasted overnight. (It is important to ensure that the patient is well hydrated before, during and after test.)

SAMPLES REQUIRED
Urine is collected in separate containers every 30 min; the time and volume are recorded. The specimen is divided to provide a 10 ml aliquot for cAMP (store at -20°C), and one for calcium, creatinine, phosphate and sodium.

PROCEDURE
The overnight urine sample should be discarded and then further samples collected as above from 0900. At t=15 min, blood is drawn for PTH, calcium, phosphate, alkaline phosphatase, albumin and sodium. At t=30 min, PTH should be given at a rate of 2 ml per minute and a second urine sample collected. Blood and urine samples are then collected every half hour (out of phase), for 2 hours.

INTERPRETATION OF RESULTS
The test is useful in distinguishing between idiopathic hypoparathyroidism and pseudohypoparathyroidism. A normal rise in cAMP in the urine after PTH administration indicates hypoparathyroidism. Patients with pseudohypoparathyroidism show no response or a diminished response depending upon the severity of the condition.

There is usually a rise in serum calcium in normal individuals and patients with idiopathic hypoparathyroidism. A blunted response is seen in patients with pseudohypoparathyroidism. A decrease in urine calcium levels may be seen in patients with idiopathic hypoparathyroidism, but not in pseudohypoparathyroidism. (For exact interpretation of urinary calcium excretion, the calcium to sodium clearance ratio should be calculated. In idiopathic hypoparathyroidism the percentage of control values is 10–60% but in pseudohypoparathyroidism is >90%.)

PHOSPHATE EXCRETION INDICES

PRINCIPLE
There is a maximal rate (transport maximum, Tm) for the active reabsorption of some solutes by the renal tubule. Abnormalities in the Tm for phosphate (TmP) may have primary causes as in familial hypophosphatemic rickets or be secondary due to the effect of parathyroid hormone. Direct assay of PTH in combination with a calcium level may obviate the need for this procedure in many cases.

MATERIALS REQUIRED
Lithium heparin containers for phosphate and creatinine estimation and urine container.

APPROXIMATE LENGTH OF TEST
One to two hours excluding overnight fast.

PATIENT PREPARATION
Overnight fast.

SAMPLES REQUIRED
After an overnight fast, collect a urine sample over 1-2 hours and a single blood sample. Assay phosphate and creatinine on each sample.

RESULTS
Calculate the following :
a) the phosphate to creatinine clearance ratio

$$C_p / C_r = \frac{P_{cr} \times U_p}{P_p \times U_{cr}}$$

where P_{cr} = plasma creatinine, P_p = plasma phosphate, U_{cr} = urine creatinine, U_p = urine phosphate, (all in mmol/l).

b) the tubular reabsorption of phosphate

$$TRP = (1-C_p/C_{cr}) \times 100$$

c) the phosphate excretion index

$$PEI = (C_p/C_{cr}) - ([0.155 \times P_p] - 0.05)$$

INTERPRETATION
In familial hypophosphatemic rickets, the TRP and TmP/GFR (which can be estimated directly or is roughly equivalent to TRP x P_p) and the plasma phosphate are low. The C_p/C_{cr} and PEI may be high.

Elevated PTH in hyperparathyroidism decreases TRP and TmP/GFR and increases C_p/C_{cr} and PEI, causing phosphaturia.

In hypoparathyroidism TRP and TmP/GFR are increased and C_p/C_{cr} and PEI are reduced.

hCG TESTS

PRINCIPLE
hCG is an LH-like compound that will stimulate testosterone production from the testes in the normal state. Testosterone is converted to DHT in the presence of normal 5α-reductase activity.

MATERIALS REQUIRED
Pharmaceutical:
• hCG. (Recombinant LH will soon be available.)
Other:
Lithium heparin containers for blood estimations of testosterone and DHT.

APPROXIMATE LENGTH OF TEST
5 days to 3 weeks (see below).

SAMPLES REQUIRED
Blood for testosterone, DHT, androstenedione, DHEA and DHEAS.

PROCEDURE
Give i.m. hCG, 1000 units for an infant and 2000 units for an older child on day 0, 1 and 2; take blood samples on days 0 and 3.

In situations of prolonged cryptorchidism, or where testicular damage is highly likely, give hCG 1000 units twice a week for 3 weeks and take blood on day 0 and 48 hours after the last injection.

INTERPRETATION
A rise in testosterone from the baseline shows intact testicular Leydig cell function. If a prolonged test produces a rise in testosterone then spontaneous puberty is possible, although surveillance will still be required and long-term ability to virilize plus fertility may still be in doubt.

A failure of a rise in DHT implies 5α-reductase deficiency. The differential rise of testosterone to DHAS and androstenedione can be used to explore defects in testosterone biosynthesis (see Chapter 6).

Appendix B

Normal Values

INTRODUCTORY NOTES

The cautions given in Chapter 8 regarding inter-assay variation, inappropriate age related values, etc, should be heeded. Ideally all values should be interpreted against a validated local range. Drugs and diet can interfere with some assays. Acute ill health, stress during the sampling procedure and prematurity can also cause variation.

Levels of steroid precursors and urinary steroid profiles, IGF-1 and IGFBP-3 levels are highly specific to the assay system used, the local population and age / pubertal status – thus normal values will not be quoted for these compounds.

Peptide hormones are given as units/litre. Standardization of biological equivalence of recombinant products to milligrams weight is currently in progress, but older human and less pure preparations are still in use to validate assays, which makes exact conversion difficult.

Normal Values

HORMONE	SI units	Conversion factor (if relevant)
ACTH (early a.m.)	2–20 pmol/l	÷ 0.22 = pg/ml
ADH	1–5 pmol/l	÷ 0.992 = pg/ml
Adrenaline		
Infant	<30 pmol/l	÷ 5.46 = ng/l
Child	<80 pmol/l	
Adult	<200 pmol/l	
Androstenedione		
Prepuberty	<3.5 nmol/l	÷ 0.0349 = ng/dl
Male	4.5–10.5 nmol/l	
Female	4–10 nmol/l	
C-peptide	20–50 nmol/l	÷ 33.3 = mg/dl
Calcitonin	<30 pmol/l	÷ 0.29 = ng/l
Cortisol		
(early a.m.)	120–660 nmol/l	÷ 28 = µg/dl
(midnight)	up to 280 nmol/l	
FSH		
Prepubertal	<3.5 IU	
Pubertal, follicular	2–7 IU	
Glucose	3.0–6.5 mmol/l	÷ 0.057 = mg/dl
GH		
(stimulated)	>20 IU/l	Approximately
(suppressed)	<2 IU/l	1mg = 3U
HbA$_1$ (assays vary)	<7%	
HbA$_{1c}$ (assays vary)	<6%	

B1 Normal values.

Normal Values contd.

HORMONE	SI units	Conversion factor (if relevant)
hCG	<5 IU/l	
17α-hydroxyprogesterone		
Males	<12 nmol/l	÷ 3.0 = µg/l
Females	<10 nmol/l	
(increased in sick and premature neonates)		
Insulin	<10 IU/l	
(interpret w.r.t. glucose in hypoglycemia)		
Lactate	<2.5 mmol/l	÷ 0.1 = mg/dl
LH		
(Prepubertal)	<2 IU	
(pubertal, follicular)	<12 IU	
(pubertal mid–cycle)	<70 IU	
Noradrenaline		
(Infant)	<100 pmol/l	÷ 5.91 = ng/l
(Older)	<900 pmol/l	
Estrogen (E2),		
(Prepubertal)	<60 pmol/l	÷ 3.67 = pg/ml
(adult male)	<250 pmol/l	
(adult female, mid cycle)	up to 1500 pmol/l	
Osmolality (plasma)	275–295 mmol/l	= mOsmol/l
Prolactin (unstressed)	< 800 pmol/l	÷ 44.4 = µg/l
Progesterone		
(prepubertal)	<1.5 nmol/l	÷ 3.18 = µg/l
(pubertal, follicular)	<5 nmol/l	
(pubertal, luteal)	15–90 nmol/l	
PTH (intact)	2–8 pmol/l	÷ 10 = ng/ml
SHBG		
(Male)	20–45 nmol/l	÷ 2.0 = µg/l
(Female)	50–80 nmol/l	
Testosterone		
(Prepubertal and female)	<1.0 nmol/l	÷ 0.035 = ng/dl
(Pubertal male, post hCG)	10–25 nmol/l	
TBG	N/A	7–17 mg/l
TSH (high sensitivity)	0.3–5.0 IU/l	
T_4 (free)	9–23 pmol/l	÷ 12.9 = ng/dl
T_4 (total)	60–160 nmol/l	÷ 13 = µg/dl
T_3 (free)	2–8.5 pmol/l	÷ 1.5 = ng/l
T_3 (total)	0.5–2.2 nmol/l	÷ 0.015 = ng/dl
Urinary free cortisol	<250 nmol/day	÷ 2.8 = µg/day
VMA (24h urine)	<40 µmol/day	÷ 5 = mg/day

Index

Numbers in bold print refer to illustrations and their captions.

3A syndrome (adrenal failure, alacrima and achalasia) 131, **1.143**

A

Aarskog syndrome
expanded finger tips/interphalangeal joints 8, **1.39**
lanugo hair **1.139**
shawl scrotum 22
Abdomen
abnormal fat **1.120**
Beckwith–Wiedemann syndrome **1.87, 3.11**
examination 19
Acanthosis nigricans 28, **1.131–1.132**
Achondroplasia 39, **2.17–2.18**
leg lengthening **2.83–2.85**
radiography **2.64**
trident hand 8, **1.35, 2.18**
Acne 91, **1.100–1.101, 4.9**
Addison's disease 131
scar pigmentation **1.130**
Adenoma
adrenal 62, **2.81**
growth–hormone producing 74
pituitary 62
Adiposity, excess 26, **1.120**
Adrenal disorders 130
Adrenal hemorrhage 130–131
Adrenal hyperplasia *see* Congenital adrenal hyperplasia
Adrenal steroid synthesis pathway **6.4**
Adrenarche 81
premature 82, 86, **1.101, 4.23**
Adrenocorticotrophic hormone (ACTH)
adrenarche 86
estimation (Synacthen test) 59, 131, 148–149
secretion 130
Alcohol
fetal alcohol syndrome *see* Fetal alcohol syndrome
ingestion 137
Aldosterone
failure of secretion 130
measurement 129–130
Androgen insensitivity syndrome **6.20–6.22, 6.34**
investigations 109
treatment 112
Androgens 81
secretion 130
Anorchia, congenital **6.40**
Anorexia nervosa **5.11–5.12**
Anthropometer 5, **1.15**
Antithyroid drugs 121–122, **7.15**
Arachnodactyly

Beals contractural 71, **3.16**
Marfan syndrome 6, **1.24–1.25, 3.15**
Arginine vasopressin (AVP) 128
assay 129
Arms 12
Arthrogryposis 6, **1.23**
Astrocytoma, intracranial **4.12**
Atrial natriuretic factor 129
Auxology 2–6
Axillary hair **1.101**

B

Back, short **2.22–2.23, 2.26–2.29**
Bardet–Biedl syndrome 25
Baroregulatory system 128
Bartter syndrome 54, 62
Beals contractural arachnodactyly 71, **3.16**
Beckwith–Wiedemann syndrome 68, **3.9–3.12**
ear crease **3.10**
facial features **3.9**
hemihypertrophy 26
umbilical hernia/organomegaly **1.87, 3.11**
Binding protein abnormalities 139–141
Body shape 26
Body mass index (Quetelet index) 5
Bone age
congenital hypothyroidism 127
early sexual development 89
hands 23, **1.104**
juvenile hypothyroidism 119
tall stature 78
Brachydactyly **1.26**
Coffin–Siris syndrome 8, **1.27**
pseudohypoparathyroidism 8, **1.28–1.29, 2.50**
Breasts
abscess, neonatal **1.90**
absent breast tissue **1.89**
central precocious puberty **4.7**
development *see* Thelarche
examination 20
gynecomastia *see* Gynecomastia
juvenile fibroadenoma **1.93**
Bruising
Cushing syndrome 29
non–accidental **1.136**
Burns, non–accidental **1.137**

C

Café–au–lait spots 26
McCune–Albright syndrome 26, **1.127**
neurofibromatosis 26, **1.125**
Calcitonin 132
Calcitriol 135
Calcium 132–136
deficiency *see* Hypocalcemia

Calcium gluconate 133
extravasation **8.16–8.17**
cAMP excretion test 150
Camptodactyly syndromes 8, **1.32**
Tel–Hashomer, scoliosis **1.85**
Candidiasis, oral 16, **1.68**
Carbimazole 121–122
Carbohydrate deficient glycoprotein syndrome 141
Cardiovascular system examination 18–19
Celiac disease 43, **2.32–2.35**
Central adrenarche stimulating hormone (CASH) 86
Central nervous system examination 23
Chemosis **7.13–7.14**
Chest examination 18
Child abuse **1.136–1.137**
Chimerism 106
Chvostek's sign 133
Cimetidine 139
Cleidocranial dysostosis **1.73–1.74**
Clinodactyly 8, **1.33**
Clitoral hypertrophy 83
Clitoroplasty 109, **6.35–6.36**
Clubbing 8, **1.41**
Coarctation of aorta 8, **2.3**
Coffin–Siris syndrome 8, **1.27**
Combined anterior pituitary function test 145–146
Congenital adrenal hyperplasia 100
acne **1.100**
hirsutism 86
treatment 91, 110–112, **6.37–6.38**
Congenital hypothyroidism 125–128, **2.42, 8.1–8.6**
Congenital lipoid hyperplasia **6.12–6.13**
Constitutional delay of growth and adolescence (CDGA) 34
Constitutional early puberty 67
Corticosteroid binding globulin (CBG) levels 139–141
Cortisol excess 137
Craniopharyngioma 128, **2.74–2.76**
papilledema **1.105**
visual fields 23, **1.107–1.108**
Craniostenosis 128
Craniosynostosis **1.55**
Cretinism (untreated congenital hypothyroidism) **2.42, 8.6**
Crohn's disease
anal signs **1.88**
fish lips **1.67**
growth failure **2.31**
Crown–rump length (sitting height) 2–3, **1.7–1.8**
Cryptorchidism 113–114, **5.3, 6.10**
Cushing syndrome 51–53
adrenal adenoma 62, **2.81**
bruising 29

buffalo hump **2.57**
causes **2.51**
facies **2.55–2.56**
hirsutism 29, **2.57**
hyperandrogenization 53
hypertension 132
iatrogenic **2.52–2.53**, **2.58**
obesity **2.54**
osteoporosis 136
pituitary adenomas 62
striae **1.140**, **2.58**
testing 59
treatment 62
Cyproterone acetate 91
Cystic fibrosis 8, **1.41**
Cystinosis **1.83**

D
DDAVP stimulation test 129, 148
De Lange syndrome **1.116**
De Morsier syndrome *see* Septo–optic
dysplasia
Dehydroepiandrosterone 86, 108
fetal adrenal cortex 141
Demeclocycline 129
Deoxycorticosterone acetate (DOCA)
131–132
Dermatoglyphics, abnormal 6, **1.16**
Desmopressin (DDAVP) test 129, 148
Dexamethasone 115
Dexamethasone suppression tests
149
Dextrose infusion 137
Diabetes insipidus 128–129
Diabetes mellitus
granuloma annulare **1.145**
hyperglycemia 138–139
intrauterine hyperinsulinemia
3.22–3.23
joint stiffness 6, **1.19**
management 139
maturity onset diabetes of youth
(MODY) 137, 139
necrobiosis lipoidica **1.144**
neonatal 138, **8.26**
oral candidiasis 16
retinopathy 138, **8.25**
Diazoxide 29, **1.138**
DIDMOAD syndrome (diabetes
insipidus, diabetes mellitus, optic
atrophy and deafness) 23
Diencephalic syndrome 44, **2.36–2.39**
Diet and laboratory tests 139
DiGeorge syndrome 16
Dihydrotestosterone 100
Dolichocephaly **1.55**
Down syndrome 13, **1.49**
Drug history 139
Dwarfism
geleophysic **1.112, 2.12–2.13**
psychosocial 54, 62, **1.136,
2.61–2.62**

Russell–Silver *see* Russell–Silver
dwarfism
Dyshormonogenesis 118, 127
Dysostosis multiplex **2.70–2.71**

E
Ears 17
abnormal helical pattern **1.76**
crease **3.10**
hairy **3.23**
low set, backward rotated **1.75**
Ectodermal dysplasia **1.69**
Ehlers–Danlos syndrome
extensible skin **1.135**
tissue paper scars **1.134**
Endocrine function tests 145–151
Endocrinopathies
artefactual 139–141
short stature 48–53
Enophthalmos **1.59**
Ergocalciferol 135
Estriol 141
Estrogen
early/excess production 82
puberty 81
replacement therapy 79, 97
Ethinylestradiol 79, 97, 98
Eunuchoid body habitus 94, **3.18, 5.1**
Examination 6–32
early sexual development 87–88
essential points **1.149**
intersex disorders 106
parents 32
short stature 56
tall stature 77
Exophthalmos **1.58, 7.13–7.14**
Eyelashes, abnormal 25, **1.116**
Eyes
blue sclerae 25, **1.114**
examination 23–25
exophthalmos **1.58, 7.13–7.14**
lens dislocation 25, **1.113**
thyrotoxicosis 122, **7.13–7.14**
see also Retina

F
Familial short stature 34
Family tree 1, **1.1**
Fatty acid oxidation disorders 137
Feet, fissued **1.143**
Fetal alcohol syndrome
hirsutism 29
typical facies 32, **1.148**
Feto–placental axis 141
Fibroadenoma, juvenile **1.93**
Finasteride 86
Fingers
expanded fingertips 8, **1.39**
fusion (syndactyly) 8, **1.30**
long, thin *see* Arachnodactyly
polysyndactyly 8, **1.31**
short *see* Brachydactyly

Fludrocortisone acetate 129, 130, 132
Follicle stimulating hormone 81, 89,
90
Forearm, limited rotation 12, **1.46**
Frusemide 129

G
Galactosemia 137
Ganglioneuromas 132
Geleophysic dwarfism **1.112,
2.12–2.13**
Gender identity (sexual identity)
101–104, **6.6**
Genitalia
abnormal 99–115
ambiguous 101–104
examination 21–22
female, early sexual development
4.25
male
central precocious puberty **4.8**
21–hydroxylase deficiency
6.31–6.32
testotoxicosis **4.21–4.22**
normal development 99–100, **6.1**
reversed **6.46**
Germinoma **2.77**
Glucagon 136
Glucocorticoid secretion 130
Glucose 136–139
Glucose tolerance tests 147
Gluten enteropathy (celiac disease)
43, **2.32–2.35**
Glycogen storage disease type–1a
2.24–2.25
Glycogen storage disorders 137
Glycosuria 138–139
Goiter 117–123, **7.1**
causes **7.2**
etiology 117–118
Graves disease **7.12**
neonatal 122, **7.16–7.17, 8.7**
palpation 17
perchlorate discharge test **8.10**
pubertal 117–118, **7.4–7.5**
radiograph **8.8**
ultrasound **8.9**
Gonadal dysgenesis 93, 103, **5.9**
Gonadotropin deficiency, isolated **6.10**
Gonadotropin releasing hormone
(GnRH) 81
analog treatment 91
test 97
Granuloma annulare **1.145**
Graves disease
exophthalmos/chemosis **7.13–7.14**
goiter **7.12**
Growth
charts ix, 5–6
failure *see* Short stature
velocity 6
Growth hormone (GH) 33

deficiency (GHD) 49–50, **2.44–2.49**
  single central incisor **1.72**
  treatment 61, 62, **2.82,
    2.86–2.87**
Growth–hormone producing
  adenoma 74
Growth hormone releasing hormone
  (GHRH) 33
Growth hormone suppression test 147
Gynecomastia 81, **6.2**
  adolescent 90–91, **1.92, 4.20**
  neonatal **1.91**
  treatment 91

H
Hair 17
  axillary **1.101**
  hirsutism *see* Hirsutism
  lanugo 29–30, **1.139, 5.2**
  loss
    hypothyroidism **1.80, 7.7–7.8**
    progeria **1.79**
    Menkes' kinky **1.78**
  pubic *see* Pubic hair
  sparse **1.77**
Hairline, low **1.52–1.53**
HAM syndrome
  (hypoparathyroidism, adrenal
  failure and moniliasis) 16
Hamartomas, hypothalamic **4.11**
Hands
  bone age estimation 23, **1.104**
  claw **1.20–1.21**
  examination 6–8
  myopathic 8, **1.34**
  trident 8, **1.35, 2.18**
Hashimoto disease 117
Head circumference 3, **1.9**
Head and neck examination 13–17
Height
  measuring 2, **1.6**
  predicted adult 23
  sitting height 2–3, **1.7–1.8**
  social class gradient 54
  target 5–6
Hemihypertrophy 26, **1.121–1.122**
Hermaphroditism
  pseudohermaphroditism *see*
    Pseudohermaphroditism
  true 103, 109, **6.7–6.8**
Hirsutism 29, 86
  Cushing syndrome 29, **2.57**
  grading **4.26**
  treatment 91
History 1, **1.2**
  early sexual development 87–88
  intersex disorders 106
  short stature 56
  tall stature 77
Holoprosencephaly **1.62–1.63**
Holt–Oram syndrome 12, **1.47**
Homocystinuria 73, **3.20**

lens dislocation 25
Hormones, normal values 153–154
Human chorionic gonadotropin
  (hCG) test 97, 151
Human growth hormone (hGH) 33
Hunter syndrome **1.21, 2.23, 2.28**
Hydrocolpos **6.49**
Hydrocortisone sodium
  hemisuccinate 132
Hydrops fetalis 137
11β–Hydroxylase adrenal hyperplasia
  88
11β–Hydroxylase deficiency 108
21–Hydroxylase deficiency 88, 89,
  100, **6.5**
  investigations 108
  male genitalia **6.31–6.32**
  masculinization **6.24–6.30**
  non–salt losing **4.15, 6.14**
  prenatal management 115
  treatment 111–112
17α–Hydroxyprogesterone 89, 90
3β–Hydroxysteroid dehydrogenase
  deficiency 108
17β–Hydroxysteroid dehydrogenase
  deficiency **6.15–6.19**
Hymen, imperforate **6.50–6.52**
Hyperaldosteronism, primary 132
Hypercalcemia 136
Hyperglycemia 138–139
Hyperinsulinemia, intrauterine 74, 78,
  137, **3.22–3.24**
Hyperlipidemia 139, **8.28**
  macroscopic **2.25**
Hypernatremia 128–132
Hyperparathyroidism, severe primary
  136
Hyperpigmentation 26–28,
  1.129–1.133
Hypertelorism **1.56**
Hypertension 18
  endocrine causes 132
Hypertrichosis 29, **1.138**
Hypoadrenalism 130
Hypoadrenocorticism 130, **8.13**
  chronic *see* Addison's disease
  secondary to insufficient ACTH
    secretion 131
  treatment 131–132
Hypoaldosteronism 130
Hypocalcemia 133
  causes **8.14**
  pseudohypoparathyroidism 51
Hypochondroplasia **2.19–2.20**
  radiography **2.65–2.66**
Hypoglycemia 137
  Beckwith–Wiedemann syndrome 68
  differential diagnosis 137
  investigations 137, 149–150, **8.24**
  micropenis 113
Hypogonadism 71–72
  eunuchoid body habitus **3.18**

hypergonadotropic 93, 97
hypogonadotropic 93, 97–98
  investigations 97–98
  Prader–Labhart–Willi syndrome
    2.10, 5.8
Hyponatremia 128–132
Hypoparathyroidism
  causes **8.15**
  HAM syndrome 16
Hypophosphatasia 31, **1.146**
Hypopituitarism
  abdominal fat, abnormal **1.120**
  enophthalmos **1.59**
  pubic hair 98
Hypospadias **6.45**
  repair 112
Hypothalamus
  dysfunction **1.115**
  hamartomas **4.11**
  tumors 74, **3.30**
Hypothyroidism **2.88**
  acquired **2.43**
  compensated 128, **8.11**
  congenital 125–128, **2.42, 8.1–8.6**
  cretinism **2.42, 8.6**
  hair loss **1.80, 7.7–7.8**
  juvenile 118–120, **7.10–7.11**
  short stature 49
  testing 59
  treatment 62, 127–128

I
Idiopathic short stature 33–34
  combined familial short stature
    and CDGA 34, **2.1**
  treatment 61
Indomethacin 62
Insulin 136
  deficiency 137
  injection sites 26, **1.118–1.119**
  resistance 137, 138–139
Insulin–like growth factor–I (IGF–I)
  33, 50
Insulin–like growth factor binding
  proteins (IGFBPs) 33
Interphalangeal joints, expanded 8,
  1.39
Intersex disorders 103–104
  history/examination 106
  investigations 106–109
  treatment 109–112
Intrauterine growth retardation
  (IUGR) 39, **2.14–2.16**
Iodine deficiency, endemic 117
Iodine[131] treatment 122
Iron deficiency 15, **1.65**
Irradiation, cranial 49–50, **2.47**

J
Joint contractures, fixed 6, **1.23**
Joints
  Aarskog syndrome 8, **1.39**

diabetes mellitus 6, **1.19**
Marfan syndrome 6, **1.17–1.18**

K

Karyotyping 106–108
Ketoconazole 91
17–Ketosteroid reductase deficiency (17β–hydroxysteroid dehydrogenase deficiency) **6.15–6.19**
Klinefelter syndrome 73
Klippel–Trenaunay–Weber syndrome **1.123, 3.21**

L

Labial adhesions 114–115, **6.53**
Lactorrhea 91, **4.33**
Langerhans' cell histiocytosis 128, **8.12**
Lanugo hair 29–30, **1.139, 5.2**
Laron syndrome 50, 59, **2.48–2.49**
treatment 62
Laurence–Moon syndrome 25, **1.111**
Leg lengthening **2.83–2.85**
Length, measuring 2, **1.5**
see also Height
Lens dislocation 25, **1.113**
Leprechaun syndrome **1.117**
Leri–Weill dyschondrosteosis 12, **1.46**
Limb hypertrophy **1.123, 3.21**
Limb segment measurement 5, **1.15**
Lipoatrophy 26, **1.118**
Lipodystrophy 26, **1.117**
Lipohypertrophy 26, **1.119**
Lips
cleft 14, **1.60**
Crohn's disease **1.67**
neuromas 15, **1.66**
Local overgrowth syndromes 73
Long bone segemental resection 79
Luteinizing hormone 81, 89, 90–91

M

McCune–Albright syndrome 83–85
café–au–lait spots 26, **1.127**
fibrous dysplasia **4.18–4.19**
treatment 91
Malignancies, screening survivors 139, **8.27**
Marfan syndrome 71, **3.13–3.15**
arachnodactyly 6, **1.24–1.25, 3.15**
high arched palate **1.64**
increased joint mobility 6, **1.17–1.18**
lens dislocation **1.113**
pectus excavatum **1.81**
sex hormone treatment 79
Marshall–Smith syndrome **3.12**
bone age 78
Maturity onset diabetes of youth (MODY) 137, 139

Mauriac syndrome **2.40–2.41**
Menarche 21
Menkes' kinky wool hair syndrome **1.78**
Metacarpal index 78
Methimazole 121–122
Methyloxidases 130
Metyrapone 29
Micropenis 112–113, **6.9–6.11**
measurement **6.39**
Midline brain structures, absent **1.110**
Midline cleft **1.62–1.63**
Mineralocorticoids
excess 132
secretion 130
Morquio syndrome (mucopolysaccharidosis type–4) **2.22, 2.29**
Mucolipidosis type–3 **1.20, 2.70–2.71**
Mucopolysaccharidosis
type–2 (juvenile Hunter syndrome) **1.21, 2.23, 2.28**
type–4 (Morquio syndrome) **2.22, 2.29**
Müllerian inhibiting factor 99, 100
deficiency **6.3**
Multiple endocrine adenomatosis (neoplasia) syndromes 123, **7.19**
investigations 78
neuromas 15, **1.66, 3.17, 3.33**
thyroid carcinoma 123
treatment 79
type–2b 71, **3.17**

N

Nails
Sotos syndrome 8, **1.42, 3.6**
Ullrich–Turner syndrome 8, **1.43–1.44**
Neck
loose skin 13, **1.49–1.50**
palpation 17
short 13, **1.54**
webbing 13, **1.51**
Necrobiosis lipoidica **1.144**
Nelson syndrome **1.129**
Neonates
pelvis **4.6**
withdrawal bleeding **4.5**
Nephrocalcinosis 133, 136
Nesidioblastosis **3.24**
Neuroblastomas 132
Neurofibromatosis
café–au–lait spots 26, **1.125**
neuromas 15, **1.126**
optic glioma **4.30–4.31**
precocious puberty **4.13–4.14, 4.30–4.31**
scoliosis **1.84**
Neuromas
multiple endocrine adenomatosis 15, **1.66, 3.17, 3.33**

neurofibromatosis 15, **1.126**
Nevi, multiple pigmented 26, **1.128**
Nevus of Ota **1.115**
Nipples, accessory 20, **1.94**
Non–salt losing 21–hydroxylase deficiency **4.15, 6.14**
Noonan syndrome 37, **2.8**
features **2.4**
neck webbing 13, **1.51**
pectus carinatum **1.82**

O

Obesity
Cushing syndrome **2.54**
growth hormone deficiency **2.46**
nutritional 67, **3.1–3.2**
Prader–Labhart–Willi syndrome **2.9**
pseudo–Cushing syndrome **2.59, 3.2**
Occipitofrontal circumference (OFC) 3, **1.9**
Optic atrophy 23, **1.106**
Optic chiasma compression **7.9**
Optic glioma **4.30–4.31**
Orchidometer **1.98**
Orchidopexy 112, 114
Organomegaly **1.87, 3.11**
Osmoregulatory system 128
Osteogenesis imperfecta
type–1 **2.69**
blue sclerae **1.114**
type–3 **2.26–2.27, 2.68**
Osteoporosis 135–136, **8.22**
Ovarian cyst, estrogen–secreting **4.16–4.17**
Ovotestis **6.7–6.8**
Oxandrolone 61, 98

P

Palate
cleft 14
panhypopituitarism **1.60**
Smith–Lemli–Opitz syndrome **1.61**
high arched **1.64**
Palms
single crease 6, **1.16**
yellow 8, **1.45**
Pancreatic endocrine dysregulation (nesidioblastosis) **3.24**
Pancreatic polypeptide 136
Panhypopituitarism **2.77, 5.13–5.14**
cleft lip/palate **1.60**
micropenis/cryptorchidism **6.9**
treatment **2.87**
Papilledema **1.105**
Parathormone 132
Parents
examination 32
history 1
Pectus carinatum **1.82**

Pectus excavatum **1.81**
Pendred syndrome 127, **8.10**
Penis
　development **1.97**
　micropenis *see* Micropenis
Perchlorate discharge test **8.10**
Phenylketonuria, undiagnosed
　maternal 32, **1.147**
Phenytoin 129
Pheochromocytomas 132
Phosphate 132–136
　excretion indices 151
Pituitary enlargement **7.9**
Pituitary gigantism 74, 78, **3.25–3.27**
　growth hormone profile **3.34**
　yellow palmar discoloration 8, **1.45**
Pituitary resistance to thyroid
　hormones (PRTH) 120
Pituitary stalk
　multiple anterior pituitary
　　hormone deficiencies **2.80**
　normal **2.79**
Pituitary tissue, ectopic **2.78**
Placental dysfunction **2.16**
Placental sulfatase deficiency 141
　lichenification **1.142**
Plasma renin activity 111, 129
Platyspondyly **2.72**
Poland sequence **1.89**
Polydipsia, primary 129
Polyglandular syndromes **7.3**
　vitiligo **1.133**
Polysyndactyly 8, **1.31**
Prader orchidometer **1.98**
Prader–Labhart–Willi syndrome 37,
　5.7
　features **2.11**
　hypogonadism **2.10**, **5.8**
　micropenis/cryptorchidism **6.11**
　obesity **2.9**
Precocious puberty *see* Sexual
　precocity
Prednisolone 132
Pregnancy
　history 1
　maternal hormone abnormalities
　　141
Pregnenolone 108
Presenting complaint 1
Priapism 79
Primary growth failure 34–41
　treatment 61
Progeria
　atrophic skin **1.141**
　hair loss **1.79**
　intrauterine growth retardation
　　2.15
Prognathism **2.23**
Prolactinomas 85, 91, **4.32**
Propanalol 121
Propylthiouracil (PTU) 121–122
Pseudo–Cushing syndrome **2.59**, **3.2**

Pseudo–hermaphroditism
　female 104, **6.23**
　male 103–104, **6.9–6.22**
Pseudohypoaldosteronism 130
Pseudohypoparathyroidism 51, 133
　abnormal helical pattern **1.76**
　brachydactyly 8, **1.28–1.29**, **2.50**
Pseudopapilledema **1.112**
PTH infusion test (cAMP excretion)
　150
Ptosis **1.57**
Pubarche, premature 82, 86, **1.101**,
　4.23
Puberty 21–22
　artifical induction 79
　early *see* Sexual precocity
　growth factor release 33
　growth spurt 21, 23, **4.10**
　hormonal changes 81
　late 93–98
Pubic hair **1.96–1.97**
　central precocious puberty **4.7**
　gonadal dysgenesis **5.9**
　hypopituitarism 98
　premature pubarche 82, 86, **1.101**,
　　4.23

Q
Quetelet index 5

R
Rachitic rosary **1.83**
Radial hypoplasia 12, **1.47**
5α–Reductase 100
Renal disease 130
Renal failure **2.30**
Renin–angiotensin–aldosterone
　system 129
Retina
　diabetic retinopathy 138, **8.25**
　dysplasia **1.109**
　storage deposits **1.112**
Retinitis pigmentosa 25, **1.111**
Rickets 134–135, **8.18–8.21**
　expanded wrist 8, **1.40**
　hypophosphataemic 40, 135, **2.21**,
　　2.67, **8.21**
　vitamin D–dependent 135,
　　8.19–8.20
Rokitansky syndrome 114
Rubinstein–Taybi syndrome
　broad thumb **1.36**
　teeth **1.69**
Russell–Silver dwarfism
　features **2.11**
　hemihypertrophy 26
　previous history of low birth
　　weight **2.14**
　sparse hair **1.77**
S
Salt losing syndromes 130–131
Salt regulation 129–132

Sclerae, blue 25, **1.114**
Scoliosis **1.84**
　laser surface mapping **1.86**
　radiograph **1.85**
　Tel–Hashomer camptodactyly **1.85**
Scrotum
　bifid 22, **1.103**
　shawl 22, 114, **1.102**, **6.41–6.44**
　trifid **6.47**
Secondary growth failure 43–54
　treatment 62
Septo–optic dysplasia (de Morsier
　syndrome) 25, 128
　absent mid–line structures **1.110**
　retinal dysplasia **1.109**
Sex chromosome disorders 99–100
Sex hormone binding globulin (SHBG)
　109, 141
Sexual development *see* Puberty
Sexual identity 101–104, **6.6**
Sexual maturation, stages 21,
　1.95–1.99
Sexual precocity 74, 81–91
　classification 82–87
　investigations 89–91
　neurofibromatosis **4.13–4.14**,
　　4.30–4.31
　optic glioma **4.30–4.31**
　pseudo–sexual precocity 83–85, 88,
　　4.15–4.22
　treatment 91
　true (central) 83, 88, **4.7–4.14**
Short stature 33–62
　aetiology 33–54
　diagnostic work–up 56–59
　disproportionate 57, **2.63–2.72**
　familial 34
　iatrogenic 54, **2.60**
　idiopathic *see* Idiopathic short
　　stature
　physiology 33
　proportionate 57, **2.73**
　proportionate with relative
　　overweight 57–59, **2.74–2.81**
　psychosocial 54, 62, **1.136**,
　　2.61–2.62
　radiographs **2.63–2.72**
　treatment 61–62
Skeletal dysplasias 39–40, **2.17–2.20**
　treatment 61, **2.83–2.85**
Skeletal maturity 23
Skin
　atrophic **1.141**
　dimpling 31, **1.146**
　dry 30–31
　examination 26–31
　extensible **1.135**
　fissured **1.143**
　fragility **1.134**
　lichenification **1.142**
　pigmentation 26–28, **1.129–1.133**
　stiffness/thickening **1.22**

Skinfold thicknesses 4, **1.10–1.13**
Smith–Lemli–Opitz syndrome **1.61**
Somatostatin 136
Somatostatin analogue treatment 79
Somatostatin release inhibiting factor
  (SRIF) 33
Sotos syndrome **3.3–3–7**, **3.12**
  deep–set nails 8, **1.42**, **3.6**
Span measurement 5, **1.14**
Spondylo–epiphyseal dysplasia 39
Spondylo–metaphyseal dysplasia 39,
  2.72
Stanazolol 109
Standard Deviation Score (Z–score) 6
Storage disorders 41
  treatment 61
Striae 30
  Cushing syndrome **1.140**, **2.58**
  idiopathic tall stature **3.32**
Stridor 133
Synacthen test 59, 131, 148–149
Syndactyly 8, **1.30**
Syndrome of inappropriate secretion
  of ADH (SIADH) 129

T
Tall stature 67–79
  aetiology 67–74
  diagnostic work–up 77–79
  familial 67
  idiopathic 67
  investigations 78
  mental retardation 68, 73, 78
  primary causes 68–73
  secondary causes 74
  treatment 79
Teeth 16–17
  abnormal shaped **1.70**
  bilirubin stained **1.71**
  delayed eruption 17, **1.73–1.74**
  peg–like **1.69**
  single central incisor **1.72**
Testicular volume 21, **1.98**
Testis determining gene 99
Testosterone
  lack of production 100
  micropenis 113
  resistance 101
  testicular 81
  therapy 79, 97–98
  intersex disorder 112
Testosterone binding protein 141
Testotoxicosis 85, **4.21–4.22**
  treatment 91
Tetany 133
Thelarche (breast development) **1.99**
  ovaries **4.27–4.29**
  premature 82, 87, **4.24**
Thromboembolism 79
Thumb
  broad **1.36**
  low set **1.38**

triphalangeal **1.37**
Thyroid carcinoma 123, **7.19**
Thyroid function tests **8.29**
Thyroid gland palpation 17
Thyroid nodules 123, **7.18**
Thyroid stimulating immunoglobulins
  (thyrotrophin receptor antibodies)
  121
Thyroidectomy, subtotal 122
Thyroiditis, autoimmune (Hashimoto
  disease) 117
Thyromegaly *see* Goiter
Thyrotoxicosis 74, 120–122, **3.28–3.29**
  exophthalmos **1.58**, **7.13–7.14**
  eye disease 122, **7.13–7.14**
  neonatal 122, **7.16–7.17**
Thyrotrophin (TSH) assays 119, 121,
  125
Thyroxine therapy 128
  juvenile hypothyroidism 120
Tissue necrosis **8.16–8.17**
Tongue
  neuromas 15, **1.66**
  smooth 15, **1.65**
Trousseau's sign 133

U
Ullrich–Turner syndrome 34
  chest, shield–like **2.3**, **2.7**
  chromosomal analysis 34
  coarctation of aorta 18, **2.3**
  features **2.4**
  final height 34
  growth hormone therapy 61, **2.82**
  high arched palate **1.64**
  hypoplastic nails 8, **1.44–1.44**
  increased carrying angle 12, **1.48**,
    2.7
  loose neck skin 13, **1.50**
  low hair line **1.52–1.53**
  nails 8, **1.43–1.44**
  neck webbing 13
  neonatal lymphedema **1.44**, **2.2**
  normal face/body type **2.5–2.6**,
    5.4–5.6
  nuchal edema 34
  osteoporosis 136
  sexual infantilism **2.7**
Umibilical hernia **1.87**, **3.11**
Uterus
  age–related changes 81, **4.1–4.4**
  cervical imprint **6.33**

V
Vagina
  atresia **6.48**
  transverse septum **6.49**
Vaginoplasty 109–110
Vas deferens 100
Vasopressin *see* Arginine vasopressin
Velocity confidence interval (CI) 6
Ventricles, clover–leaf **1.63**

Very long chain fatty acids 131
Virginal breast hypertrophy (juvenile
  fibroadenoma) **1.93**
Virilization, maternal 141
Visual fields 23, **1.107–1.108**
Vitamin D (calciferol)
  metabolism 132
  supplements 133, 135
Vitiligo 28, **1.133**, **5.10**, **7.6**

W
Water deprivation test 148
Water regulation 128–129
Weaver syndrome **3.8**, **3.12**
Weight, measuring 2, **1.3–1.4**
Wllllams syndrome 136, **8.23**
Wilms' tumor 26
Wolffian duct 100
Wrist
  bone age estimation 23, **1.104**
  expansion, rickets 8, **1.40**

X
XX male 99, 108, **6.2**
XY karyotype 108–109
XYY syndrome 73, **3.19**

Z
Z–score 6